KU-161-867

Praise for *Relax and Renew*

"I welcome this fine book to our anxious and weary world. We all need the wisdom it contains. . . . Restorative yoga has been helpful for my patients with such diverse conditions as back pain, neck pain, high blood pressure, asthma, migraine and tension headaches, stress-related diseases, chronic fatigue, chronic obstructive pulmonary disease, and cancer."

MARY PULLIG SCHATZ, M.D., Author of *Back Care Basics* and *Relaxation Basics*

"In *Relax and Renew,* Judith Lasater writes with insight and clarity about a subject she loves: restorative yoga. These techniques will help you ease stress and live well."

DEAN ORNISH, M.D., Author of *Dr. Dean Ornish's Program for Reversing Heart Disease; Eat More, Weigh Less;* and *Stress, Diet, and Your Heart*

"Judith Lasater brings wisdom and experience to this remarkable book. Her suggestions for menstruation, pregnancy, and menopause are invaluable for women today."

SADJA GREENWOOD, M.D., Author of *Menopause, Naturally*

"This book can help anyone develop and deepen the practice of yoga, and use it in the work of healing not only one's body, but one's life. The detailed recommendations for practicing the various postures are extremely valuable. Restorative yoga can be a gateway to deep relaxation and the cultivation of mindfulness. Enter, enter!"

JON KABAT-ZINN, UMMC Center for Mindfulness in Medicine, Health Care, and Society, Author of *Wherever You Go, There You Are* and *Full Catastrophe Living*

"*Relax and Renew* is a major contribution to the study of relaxation. It offers you skillful ways to mind the body and mend the mind."

JOAN BORYSENKO, PH.D., Author of *Minding the Body, Mending the Mind* and *The Power of the Mind to Heal*

RELAX AND RENEW

Books by Judith Hanson Lasater

Living Your Yoga (2000)

30 Essential Yoga Poses (2003)

Yoga for Pregnancy (2004)

Yoga Abs (2005)

A Year of Living Your Yoga (2006)

Yogabody (2009)

What We Say Matters (2009)

Relax and Renew (2nd edition, 2011)

Restore and Rebalance (2017)

RELAX AND RENEW

Restful Yoga for Stressful Times

Judith Hanson Lasater, Ph.D., P.T.

Foreword by
Mary Pullig Schatz, M.D.

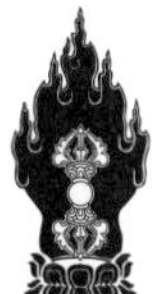

Shambhala • Boulder • 2011

Shambhala Publications, Inc.
2129 13th Street
Boulder, Colorado 80302
www.shambhala.com

A Rodmell Press book

© 1995, 2011 by Judith Hanson Lasater, Ph.D., P.T.
Interior photographs © 1995 by Fred Stimson
Cover photograph © 2005 David Martinez Inc.

All rights reserved. No part of this book may be reproduced in any form or by any means, electronic or mechanical, including photocopying, recording, or by any information storage and retrieval system, without permission in writing from the publisher.

14 13 12 11 10 9 8

Printed in United States of America

♾ This edition is printed on acid-free paper that meets the American National Standards Institute Z39.48 Standard.

♻ Shambhala Publications makes every effort to print on recycled paper. For more information please visit www.shambhala.com.

Shambhala Publications is distributed worldwide by Penguin Random House, Inc., and its subsidiaries.

Editors: Holly Hammond, Linda Cogozzo
Indexer: Ty Koontz
Design: Gopa & Ted2, Inc.
Photographer: Fred Stimson
Cover Photographer: David Martinez Inc.
Illustrator: Halstead Hannah

Text set in Meridien LT

Library of Congress Cataloging-in-Publication Data
Lasater, Judith. Relax and renew: restful yoga for stressful times/Judith Lasater; foreword by Mary Pullig Schatz. 1st ed. Berkeley, CA: Rodmell Press, 1995.
xvi, 240 p.: ill.; 26 cm.
RA781.7.L37 1995
ISBN 978-0-9627138-4-2 (pbk.: first edition)
ISBN 978-1-930485-29-7 (pbk.: second edition)

Grateful acknowledgment is made to the following for permission to reprint previously published material:

Carol Publishing Group: Excerpt from *The Wellness Book* by Herbert Benson, M.D., Eileen M. Stuart, and the Staff of the Mind/Body Medical Institute of New England Deaconess Hospital and Harvard Medical School; copyright © 1992 by The Mind/Body Medical Institute. Reprinted by permission of Carol Publishing Group.

Farrar, Straus & Giroux, Inc.: Excerpt from *Sappho: A Garland* translated by Jim Powell; copyright © 1993 by Jim Powell. Reprinted by permission of Farrar, Straus & Giroux, Inc.

Times Books: Excerpt from *Living Beyond Limits* by David Spiegel, M.D.; copyright © 1993 by David Spiegel, M.D. Reprinted by permission of Times Books, a division of Random House, Inc., New York.

In addition, we thank:

KD Dance: For permission to use their handloomed knitwear in the interior photographs; (800) 443-1371, www.kddance.com.

Hugger-Mugger Yoga Products: For permission to use their props in the photographs; (800) 473-4888, www.huggermugger.com.

Marie Wright Yoga Wear: For permission to use their unitard in the cover photograph; (800) 217-0006, www.mariewright.com.

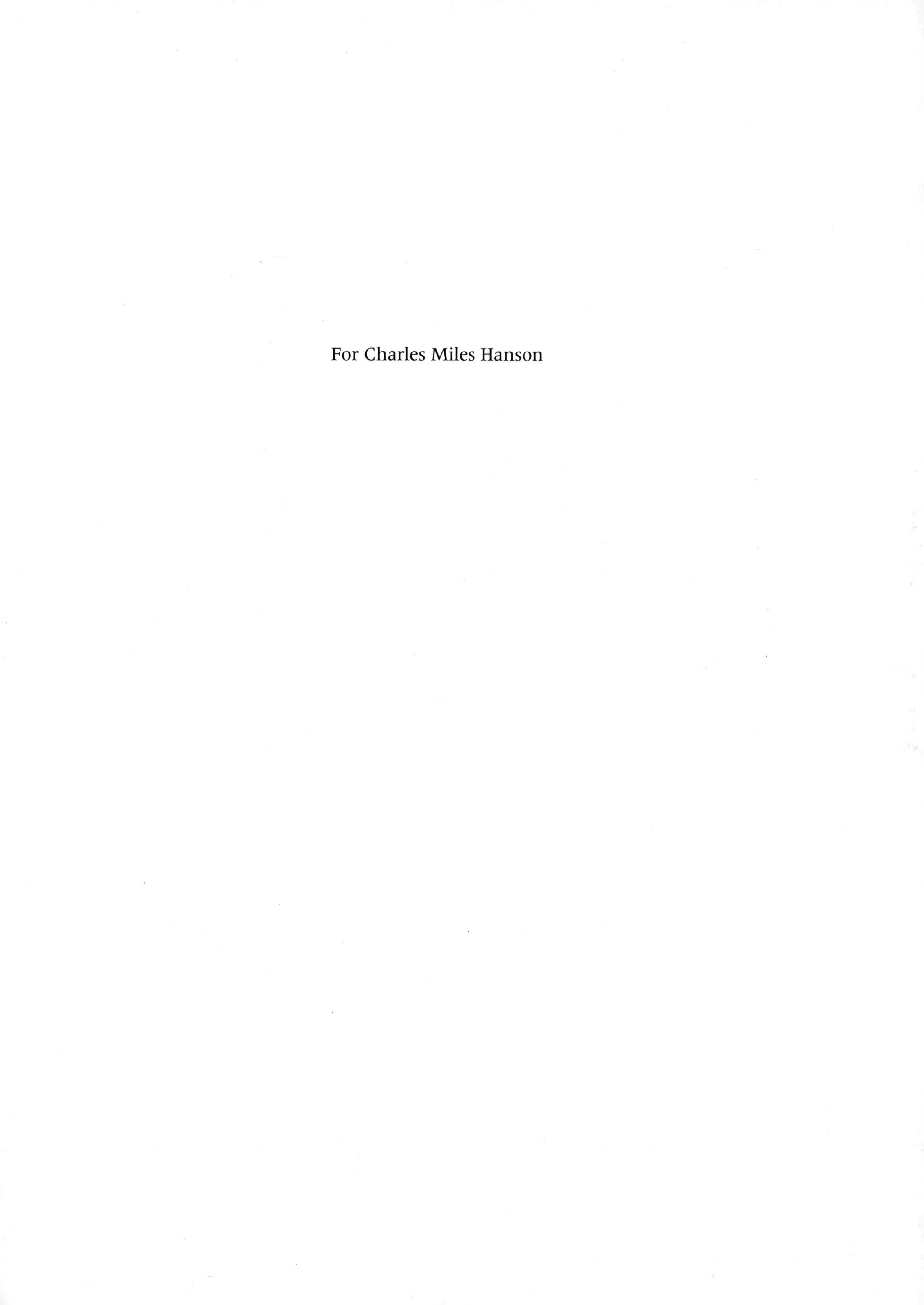

For Charles Miles Hanson

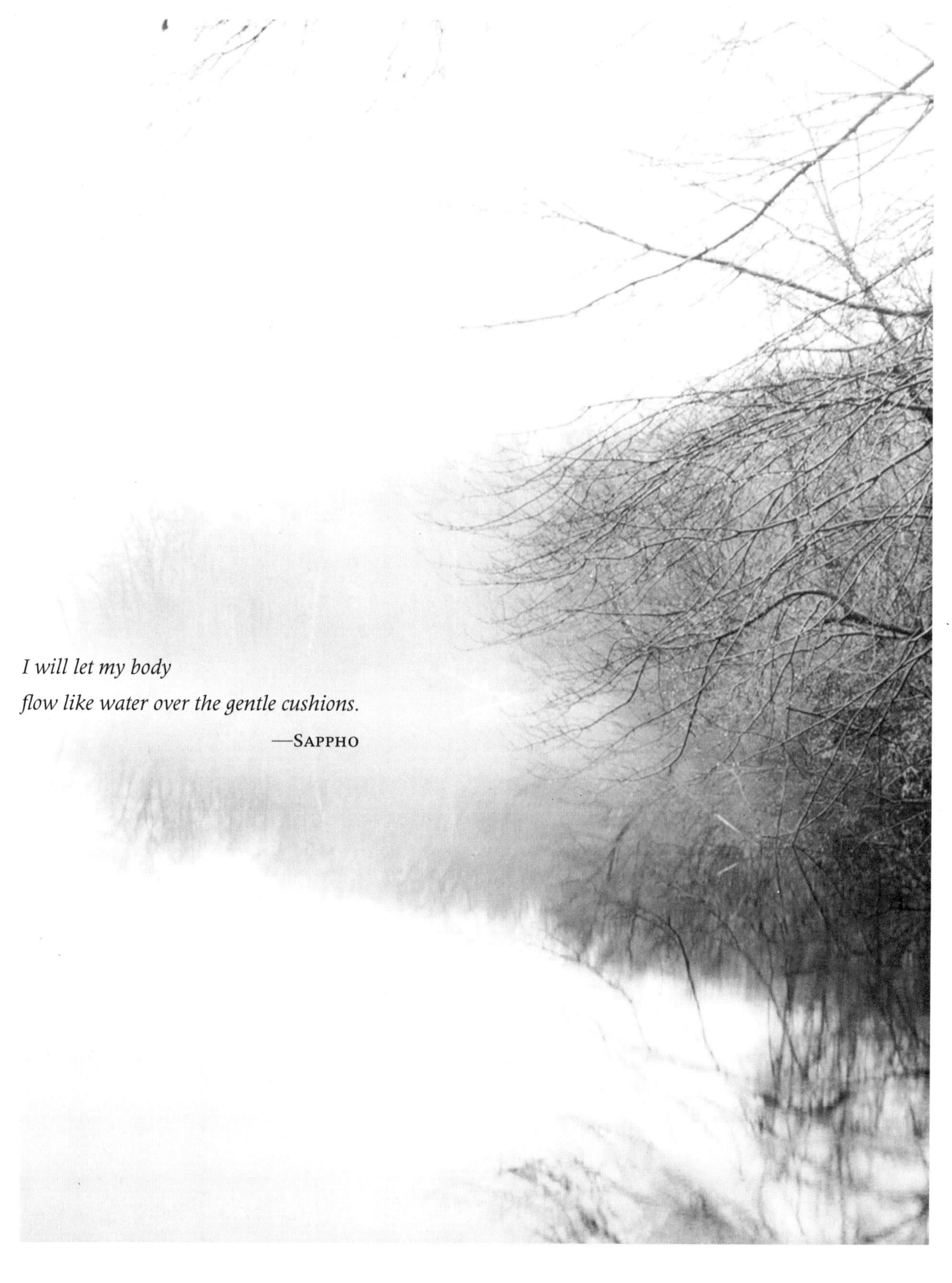

I will let my body
flow like water over the gentle cushions.

—Sappho

CONTENTS

ACKNOWLEDGMENTS

LIKE MOST PROJECTS in life, writing a book is a team effort. I gratefully acknowledge the members of my team:

My children, Miles, Kam, and Elizabeth, for their love and willingness to make room in their lives for "Mom's book." I also appreciate their computer expertise and frequent help for their "low-tech" Mom;

My daughter-in-law, Liz, for her good nature, for supporting Miles, and for caring about our family;

My grandson, Owen, for his enchanting laugh and love of life;

B.K.S. Iyengar, for his teachings. I have gained tremendous insight from his work and an invaluable foundation in yoga;

My students, who have inspired me to teach and write about yoga through the years;

Linda Cogozzo, my editor, for her ability to see the book in a new way, over and over again;

Kathy Glass, Holly Hammond, Katherine L. Kaiser, and Patricia Kaminski, for their valuable editorial assistance;

Mary Pullig Schatz, M.D., who gave of her time and expertise to write the foreword;

Gopa & Ted2, Inc., whose designs gave life to the second editon of this book;

Fred Stimson, for his sensitive and skillful asana and nature photography;

Amanda Stimson, for her expert assistance and generous spirit;

David Martinez, for his simply beautiful cover photograph;

Halstead Hannah, who brought elegant clarity to the illustrations;

Theresa Elliott, Carol Nelson, Richard Rosen, and Carol Wong, who modeled for the cover and interior photographs with patience and good humor;

Sara Chambers, Tricia Kaye, and Ray Kerr, who helped with some of the production details for the photo shoot;

And finally, Donald Moyer and Linda Cogozzo, who are friends and publishers extraordinaire.

FOREWORD

I WELCOME THIS FINE BOOK to our anxious and weary world. We all need the wisdom it contains. In *Relax and Renew,* Judith Lasater presents a synthesis of ancient knowledge and modern science, informed by her experiences as a wife, mother, yoga teacher, and physical therapist. She gives sound advice to the caregivers of the world: It is imperative that we take care of ourselves, otherwise life's stresses will make us unable to care for those who depend on us. Then she shows us, step-by-step, how to make the most of precious private time by doing less through the techniques of restorative yoga. By so doing, we can release ourselves from the destructive forces of chronic stress.

Restorative yoga has been an important part of my professional and personal life for many years. I first became aware of it while studying with B.K.S. Iyengar at the Ramamani Iyengar Memorial Yoga Institute in Pune, India. In addition to yoga classes that focused on active yoga postures for healthy people, Mr. Iyengar conducted special therapeutic classes for those with a variety of ailments. Many had been referred to these classes by their physicians. I was amazed to see students of all ages practicing this entirely different form of yoga. Each had a personalized series of passive poses, supported by various combinations of pillows, folded or rolled blankets, and odd pieces of furniture. Needless to say, my medical curiosity was thoroughly aroused. On subsequent visits, I interviewed these students and followed them through their routines.

During one visit, I was having severe pelvic pain from endometriosis. Mr. Iyengar gave me a "yoga prescription" very similar to the Moon Club series (chapter 12) in *Relax and Renew.* It worked wonders and helped me get through a difficult phase in my life. As I experienced the effects of these soothing, quieting poses on my own body, I realized that their power came from helping my own internal healing processes to work—healing processes that had been overwhelmed by stress and disease.

Since then, I have used various combinations of active yoga and restorative yoga for managing my own stress, recovering from surgery, and dealing with the menopausal transition. Professionally, restorative yoga has been helpful for my patients with such diverse conditions as back pain, neck pain, high blood pressure, asthma, migraine and tension headaches, stress-related diseases, chronic fatigue, chronic obstructive pulmonary disease, and cancer.

Judith Lasater has brought restorative yoga to many yoga students and teachers through her numerous classes, workshops, and magazine articles over the years. With *Relax and Renew,* even greater numbers of women and men will have the opportunity to learn from her. Yoga teachers and students will find her approach an important addition to their teaching and practice. Readers unfamiliar with yoga will discover a gentle introduction to time-honored techniques that help people take better care of themselves.

MARY PULLIG SCHATZ, M.D.
Author of *Back Care Basics* and *Relaxation Basics*

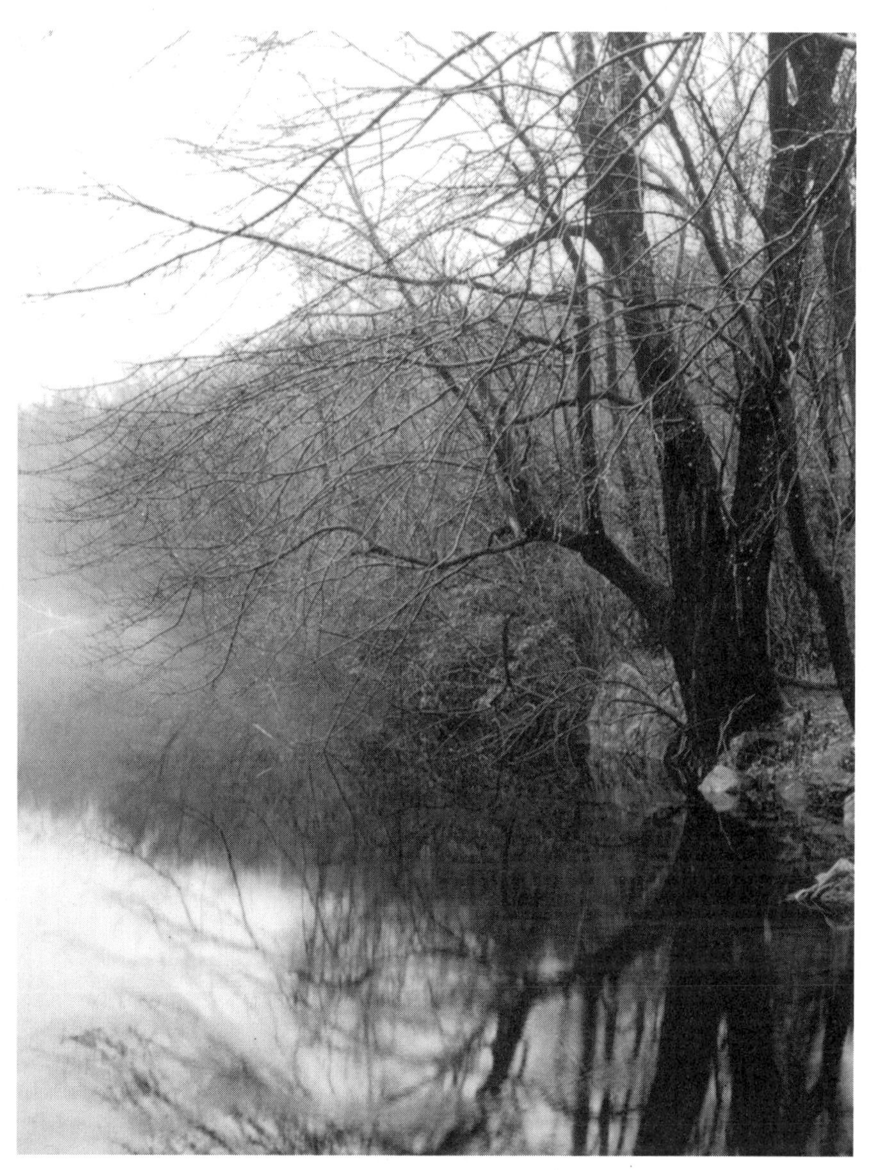

PART ONE: RELAX AND RENEW

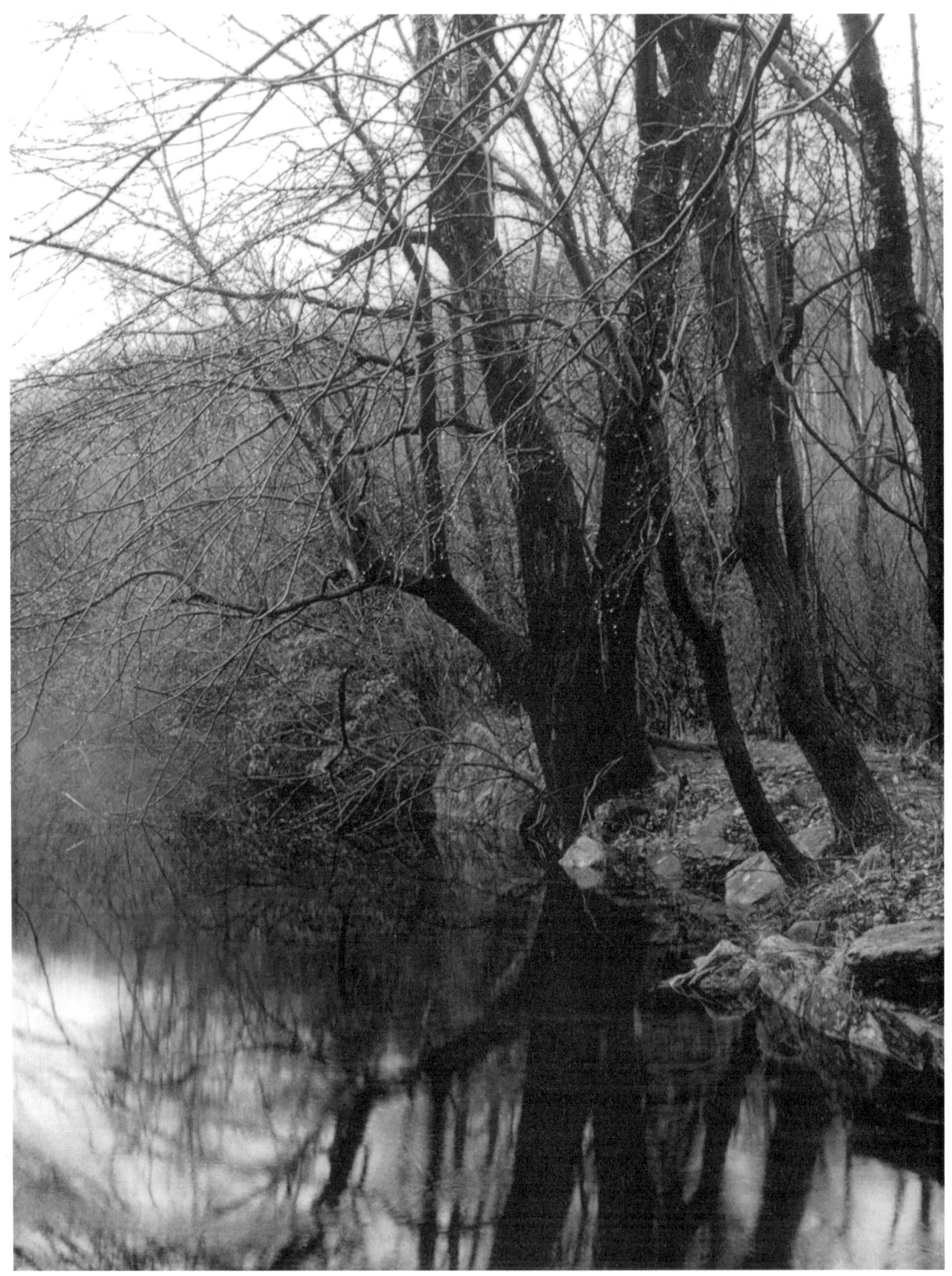

CHAPTER ONE

RESTORATIVE YOGA

The Antidote to Stress

TAKING TIME OUT each day to relax and renew is essential to living well. This book presents nurturing physical postures based on yoga. When practiced regularly, they will help you to heal the effects of chronic stress in as little as five minutes a day.

Anthropologists tell us the body that experiences stress has not changed much over the millions of years of being human. Our ancestors had the same anatomical and physiological characteristics as we who drive freeways and communicate via the information superhighway. We have an ancient body subjected to a modern problem: living with chronic stress.

At one time, stress was a term used chiefly by physiologists who measured its effects in their laboratories. Today the term is used in common parlance. "I'm stressed out" is a familiar idiom describing how a life lived on overload affects health, sexual function and reproduction, relationships, job performance, athletic performance, and, most important, our sense of self. The effects of stress have reached epidemic proportions in our lives, and stress-related diseases have become a medical specialty.

Sometimes the effects of stress present themselves during milestone life events: marriage, birth of a child, getting a new job, or death of a loved one. Other times it's the little things that get us as we try to juggle the myriad responsibilities of job and family. Regardless of the trigger, stress is often accompanied by one or more negative effects—impatience, frustration, irritation, anger, muscle tension, headache, indigestion, or poor elimination. One thing is certain: The more stress we experience, the more its effects compound within us. When stress becomes chronic, a residue builds up in the body that can lead to disease.

Stress Can Make You Sick

Don't worry about things you cannot alter.
—Catherine the Great

Stress begins with a physiological response to what your body-mind perceives as life-threatening. For our ancestors, this may have been defending against the aggression of a hungry animal. For modern-day humans, this may be living with the fear of losing a job in a sagging economy, or the health crisis of a family member.

Whatever the stressor, the mind alerts the body that danger is present. In response, the adrenal glands, located above the kidneys, secrete catecholamine hormones. These adrenaline and noradrenalin hormones act upon the autonomic nervous system, as the body prepares for fight or flight. Heart rate, blood pressure, mental alertness, and muscle tension are increased. The adrenal hormones cause metabolic changes that make energy stores available to each cell, and the body begins to sweat. The body also shuts down systems that are not a priority in the immediacy of the moment, including digestion, elimination, growth, repair, and reproduction.

These adaptive responses have been positive for the survival of the human race over thousands of years. For our ancestors, a stressful situation usually resolved itself quickly. They fought or they ran, and if they survived, everything returned to normal. The hormones were used beneficially, the adrenal glands stopped producing stress hormones, and systems that were temporarily shut down resumed operation.

To our detriment, modern people are often unable to resolve our stress so directly, and we live chronically stressed as a result. Still responding to the fight-or-flight response, the adrenals continue to pump stress hormones. The body does not benefit from nutrition because the digestion and elimination systems are slowed down. Even sleep is disturbed by this agitated state.

In a chronically stressed condition, quality of life, and perhaps life itself, is at risk. The body's capacity to heal itself is compromised, either inhibiting recovery from an existing illness or injury, or creating a new one, including high blood pressure, ulcers, back pain, immune dysfunction, reproductive problems, and depression. These conditions add stress of their own, and the cycle continues.

The Relaxation Solution

The antidote to stress is relaxation. To relax is to rest deeply. This rest is different from sleep. Deep states of sleep include periods of dreaming, which increase muscular tension, as well as other physiological signs of tension. Relaxation is a state in which there is no movement, no effort, and the brain is quiet.

Common to all stress reduction techniques is putting the body in a comfortable position, with gentle attention directed toward the breath. Do these techniques really work? Scientists have researched the effects of relaxation and report measurable benefits, including reduction in muscle tension and improved circulation.

Among the first to study relaxation was Edmund Jacobson, M.D. In 1934, he wrote *You Must Relax* about the benefits of his progressive relaxation techniques. He reported success in using his approach to treat high blood pressure, indigestion, colitis, insomnia, and what he called "nervousness."[1]

One of the foremost writers and researchers in the field of stress reduction today is Herbert Benson, M.D., who coined the phrase "relaxation response" to describe the physiological and mental responses that occur when one consciously relaxes. In *The Wellness Book,* he defines the relaxation response as "a physiological state characterized by a slower heart rate, metabolism, rate of breathing, lower blood pressure, and slower brain wave patterns."[2]

David Spiegel, M.D., author of *Living Beyond Limits,* reports, "In medicine, we are learning that physical problems such as high blood pressure and heart disease can be influenced by psychological interventions such as relaxation training. Indeed, the Food and Drug Administration issued a report recommending these non-drug approaches as the treatment of choice for milder forms of hypertension. Mind and body are connected and must work together, and this should be a powerful asset in treating medical illness."[3]

Even adults have numerous possibilities for change.
—Don Johnson

Indeed, body and mind are connected. The medical specialty called psychoneuroimmunology is an interdisciplinary field that studies the interaction between psychological processes and our nervous and immune systems. This field understands that the health of the psyche is reflected in, and partly created by, the health of the body, and vice versa.[4]

Among those whose scientific study supports the body-mind connection is Dean Ornish, M.D., author of *Dr. Dean Ornish's Program for Reversing Heart Disease.* He studied those with atherosclerotic heart disease and concluded that daily periods of relaxation are essential in preventing further deterioration. Ornish also created a unique lifestyle program that includes diet, yoga, and meditation.[5]

Restorative Yoga

Good judgment comes from experience, but experience comes from bad judgment.
—ANONYMOUS

The word *yoga* comes from Sanskrit, the scriptural language of ancient India, and means "to yoke" or "to unite." Dating back to the Indus Valley civilization of 2000 to 4000 B.C.E., yoga practices are designed to help the individual feel whole. Ancient yoga texts present teachings that include the physical, mental, and spiritual dimensions of the practitioner. The physical aspects—poses (*asana*) and breathing techniques (*pranayama*)—are the most popular of yoga teachings in the West.

Typically a yoga class or personal practice session begins with a series of active poses followed by a brief restorative pose. In this book, I'll place the entire focus of practice on the restorative poses. The development of these poses is credited to B.K.S. Iyengar, of Pune, India. Author of the contemporary classic *Light on Yoga* and numerous other books, Iyengar has been teaching yoga for seventy-five years.[6] Widely recognized as a worldwide authority, he is one of the most creative teachers of yoga today.

Iyengar's early teaching experience showed him how pain or injury can result from a student straining in a yoga pose. He experimented with props—simple tools used to modify poses so the student could practice without strain. Iyengar also explored how these modified poses could help people recover from illness or injury. It is because of his creativity that the restorative poses in this book—most of which have been developed or directly inspired by him—are such powerful tools to reduce stress and restore health.

I often refer to restorative yoga poses as "active relaxation." By supporting the body with props, we alternately stimulate and relax the body to move toward balance. Some poses have an overall benefit. Others target an individual part, like the lungs or heart. All create specific physiological responses that are beneficial to health and can reduce the effects of stress-related disease.

In general, restorative poses are for those times when you feel weak, fatigued, or stressed from your daily acitivities. They are especially beneficial for the times before, during, and after major life events: death of a loved one, change of job or residence, marriage, divorce, major holidays, and vacations. In addition, you can practice the poses when ill or recovering from illness or injury.

How Restorative Yoga Works

Restorative poses relieve the effects of chronic stress in several ways. First, the use of props as described in this book provides a completely supportive environment for total relaxation.

Second, each restorative sequence is designed to move the spine in all directions. These movements illustrate the age-old wisdom of yoga that well-being is enhanced by a healthy spine. Some of the restorative poses are back bends, while others are forward bends. Additional poses gently twist the column both left and right.

Third, a well-sequenced restorative practice also includes an inverted pose, which reverses the effects of gravity. This can be as simple as putting your legs on a bolster or pillow, but the effects are quite dramatic. Because we stand or sit most of the day, blood and lymph fluid accumulate in the lower extremities. By changing the relationship of the legs to gravity, fluids are returned to the upper body, and heart function is enhanced.

Psychobiologist and yoga teacher Roger Cole, Ph.D., consultant to the University of California, San Diego, in sleep research and biological rhythms, has done preliminary research on the effects of inverted poses. He found that they dramatically alter hormone levels, thus reducing brain arousal, blood pressure, and fluid retention. He attributes these benefits to a slowing of heart rate and dilation of the blood vessels in the upper body due to reversing the effects of gravity.[7]

Fourth, restorative yoga alternately stimulates and soothes the organs. For example, by closing the abdomen with a forward bend and then opening it with a back bend, the abdominal organs are squeezed, forcing the blood out, and then opened, so fresh blood returns to soak the organs. With this movement of blood comes the enhanced exchange of oxygen and waste products across the cell membrane.

Finally, yoga teaches that the body is permeated with energy. *Prana,* the masculine energy, resides above the diaphragm, moves upward, and controls respiration and heart rate. *Apana,* the feminine energy, resides below the diaphragm, moves downward, and controls the function of the abdominal organs. Restorative yoga balances these two aspects of energy so the practitioner is neither overstimulated nor depleted.

How to Use This Book

I know that you are eager to begin, but it is a good idea to read chapters 2 and 3 before proceeding with practice. They contain information designed to make your experience of restorative yoga a safe and satisfying one. Chapter 2 answers those questions most often asked by my students about how to practice, including general cautions. Chapter 3 gives you step-by-step information on props; you'll learn what they are, where they go, how to fold blankets, and more.

There are no riches above a sound body.
—**Ecclesiastes 30:16**

Chapters 4 and 5 are the core of restorative practice as presented in this book, introducing Basic Relaxation Pose, the Centering Breath, and the Relax and Renew series. Chapter 6 offers practice alternatives for those inevitable days when time is tight. There's even a practice for you to do at work.

> A wish to be well is part of becoming well.
> —Seneca

Chapters 7 through 11 present restorative yoga solutions for the stresses of life: back pain, headaches, insomnia, breathing difficulties, and jet lag.

Chapters 12 through 14 offer restorative yoga for women's needs during menstruation, pregnancy, and menopause. This information is also insightful for their partners who want to understand more about these special times.

Chapters 15 through 18 emphasize techniques to take your yoga practice into your daily life of breathing, standing, sitting, and being.

The appendix offers resources and recommended reading, including some of the best health and relaxation information and tools I know about.

The poses in each series are presented in a specific sequence that gradually moves you toward deeper states of relaxation. To experience maximum benefit, practice them in the order given. The effects of each series are cumulative. I have taken into consideration that you might not have time to practice an entire series, so the programs in chapter 6 are offered as an alternative to chapter 5. And at the end of chapters 7 through 14 are shorter programs using poses in the series. In any case, if you have only five minutes, practice a variation of Basic Relaxation Pose appropriate for you.

Each pose contains several sections of information. I recommend that you read the instructions completely for each pose the first few times you practice until you become familiar with what is being asked of you.

- Props and Optional Props are presented like recipes in a cookbook to help you assemble what you need to begin. Feel free to use things you have around the house. You can always refer to chapter 3 for helpful suggestions.
- Setting Up explains how to position yourself and the props. In some cases, a pose is presented in more than one chapter. To read the full description, you will sometimes be asked to refer to a previous page, although essential information is usually repeated, and changes to the basic pose are clearly presented. As you practice, these repeated poses will become familiar to you.
- Being There offers gentle guidance for spending time in the pose.

- Coming Back details how long to stay in the pose and how to come out safely.
- Benefits explains what the pose will do for you.
- Cautions lets you know when not to do the pose.

Reaching Out: Finding a Yoga Teacher

While restorative poses are simple and straightforward, you may decide to seek the guidance of a teacher or the camaraderie of a yoga class. Choose a teacher with care (see Resources). A good teacher is knowledgeable, supportive, and respectful. Different teachers have different approaches to yoga and, unlike other professions, yoga teachers are not required to be accredited. Here are important things to consider when looking for a teacher:

- Ask questions. Not all yoga teachers are trained in restorative yoga. Call ahead to inquire about training and approach to teaching.
- Observe a class before you take one. Most teachers welcome observers. Use this time to assess the teacher's ability, relationship with students, and approach to relaxation.
- You are the best authority about your body. A good teacher is authoritative, not authoritarian. Avoid those who insist that you try things you feel you are not ready for, or who want you to stay in a pose even when it is uncomfortable for you.
- Follow your heart. There is more to yoga than poses. Study with a teacher you trust and feel good about.

Carry On

Learning to relax is at the heart of living well, but opening your life to include a regular restorative practice is a challenge. It may be difficult to find time in an already busy schedule. Sometimes your practice will not be satisfying, and you'll wonder what good it's doing. Your mind will protest that you're wasting your time when there is so much else to be done. It is at these moments when it is most important to continue. Consider your practice an experiment that you carry out with the finest instruments at your command: your body, your breath, and your mind.

I am worn to a raveling.
—Beatrix Potter

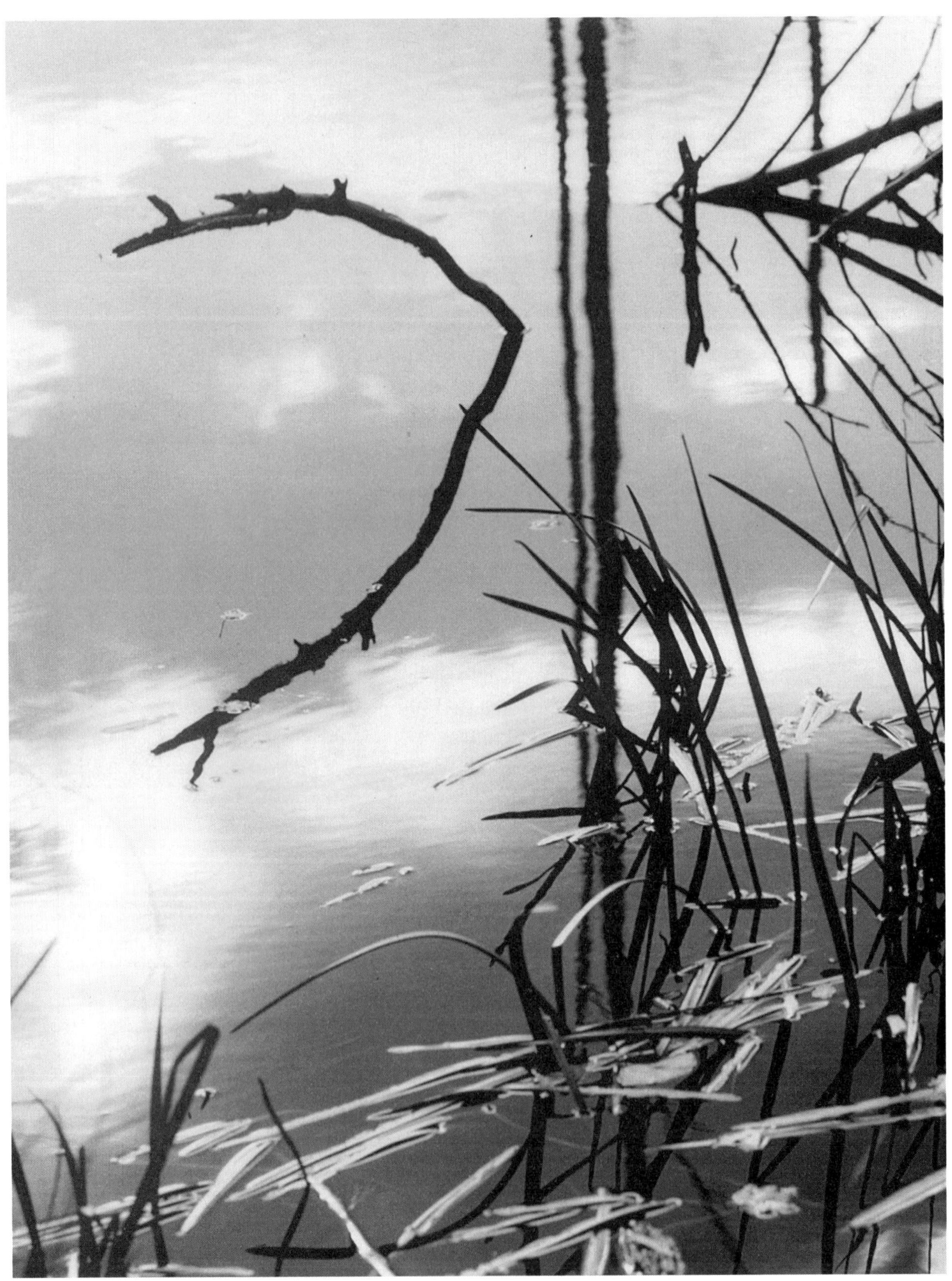

CHAPTER TWO

GETTING STARTED

It's Easier Than You Think

■ ■ ■

WELCOME TO THE practice of restorative yoga. Most of us lead lives that reinforce our working at fast-forward speed and then collapsing in exhaustion. We have very few habits that encourage balance between these two extremes. I call this balance point the art of being relaxed. Restorative yoga poses will teach you how. Think of them as taking a short holiday right in your bedroom or living room, and this book as your passport.

Before you begin, familiarize yourself with the information in this chapter and in chapter 3. Based on questions my yoga students have asked over the years, I have tried to anticipate those you might have about getting started. The care and attention you bring to these first steps—from finding the right place to practice, to folding blankets, to adjusting props—will make your experience truly restorative.

Gentle is that gentle does.
—English Proverb

- **I don't have enough time as it is. How can I add yoga to my life?** So often we feel intimidated by doing something new or something that requires more of us when we are already stressed out. For the next three days, write down what you do in half-hour increments, from 7 A.M. through 9:30 P.M. This exercise will help you discover how you spend your time. You may uncover five minutes, fifteen minutes, or maybe more time that you can give to your restorative yoga practice.

- **Where do I begin?** Do what is possible, and be consistent. Practicing just one pose a day is better than a long practice every now and then. The more regularly you practice, the more you will feel the effects.

  If you are new to yoga, begin with a 5- to 15-minute practice of Basic Relaxation Pose, as described in chapter 4. Add poses as you feel ready. You can expand to include some or all of the series in chapter 5. For days when time is at a premium, you can practice one of the three shorter routines from chapter 6.

  If you already have an established yoga practice or want to combine restorative poses with the practice of more active yoga poses, choose one or two suitable poses to add to your daily routine. You may want to devote one day's practice each week to restorative poses. Some individuals find Sunday a perfect day to practice them because they have a more relaxed schedule on that day.

- **When should I practice?** You will feel some benefit no matter what time of day you practice these poses. In general, choose a time when you know you will feel the least rushed. If your time is more flexible, experiment with what feels the most natural for your body's rhythms. Many students choose to practice in the morning. They find that if they wait until later, they are too tired and fall asleep in the poses. Others prefer practicing in the late afternoon, a time when restorative practice provides a rest after the demands of the day and prepares you to start the evening refreshed.

- **Where should I practice?** Choose a comfortable, quiet area. If the only place you have is filled with the demands of daily life, make it as stress-free as possible. If it's at work, let your colleagues know you're having a relaxation break and don't want to be disturbed; close the door, unplug the telephone, turn off your computer, and dim the lights.

  The floor should be clean and even; practicing on a rug, carpet, or folded blanket is fine. If you tend to get cold, have an extra blanket nearby to cover yourself. A favorite quilt or thermal blanket works well.

- **What should I wear? What if I'm practicing at my office?** The models in the photographs are dressed to show the maximum amount of detail for each pose. However, it is not necessary that you buy costly exercise gear. Choose clothing that allows you to move freely and keeps you comfortably warm. In general, you can wear your socks. For some poses, you will need to remove them, but this will be detailed later.

  If you are practicing at your office, take off your necktie, undo the top button on your shirt or blouse and any buttons at your wrists or waist, loosen your belt, and remove your shoes if it's appropriate to do so. No matter where you practice, remove your eye glasses or contact lenses and your wristwatch.

- **Can I eat before practice?** Wait at least two hours after eating before you practice. Some people prefer even more time. Allowing some time for digestion will decrease agitation from within. The most important thing is that you feel comfortable and can breathe easily.

- **I have difficulty getting down to and up from the floor to practice. What should I do?** Lean on a stable chair or another piece of furniture for support to help you get down and up. If you still encounter difficulty, practice on your bed, sofa, reclining chair, or chaise lounge. (See chapter 17 for instructions on how to relax in a chair.)

- **How do I know I'm doing it right?** The answer is in how you feel. While you are in a pose, allow your attention to move inward, and notice how your body responds. All the poses should feel comfortable. Take the time you need to adjust your props so you can really relax.

The greatest thing in the world is for a man to know how to be himself.
—Montaigne

- **What should I do if I experience pain or discomfort in the pose?** If you feel pain in any pose, come out as described in the Coming Back section of each pose. Reread the instructions; add or subtract props, modify their sizes, and experiment with placement. Try the pose again. In many cases, I offer you practice alternatives. For example, if you experience lower back pain in Basic Relaxation Pose (chapter 4), try Side-Lying Relaxation Pose (chapter 13). If pain or discomfort persist, consult your health care professional on how and when to resume practice of the pose.

- **How should I breathe?** In general, allow your breath to move slowly and smoothly through the nose, with mouth closed. In some poses, I guide you through a specific breathing awareness practice called the Centering Breath.

- **Is it okay to listen to music while I practice?** Many people enjoy listening to soothing music while practicing restorative poses. While there is nothing intrinsically wrong with this, my preference is for you to practice in a quiet space. I encourage you to do so for two reasons. First, it is easy to get carried away in reverie by the music and not be aware of your body, breath, and mind as they exist in the present moment. Second, so much of daily living is bombarded by noise. Restorative practice gives us the opportunity to simplify and learn to do one thing at a time.

- **How will I know when to come out of the pose?** Check the Coming Back section of each pose. It will tell you how long to stay and how to come out of the pose safely. You can always set an alarm clock or timer and let it keep the time so you can relax. (If the sound of the clock or the alarm is disturbing, place a pillow over it before you lie down.) Come out of each pose slowly to maintain a physical feeling of relaxation.

General Cautions for Practice

Only in growth, reform, and change, paradoxically enough, is true security to be found.
—Anne Morrow Lindbergh

The restorative poses are usually experienced as so gentle that it is easy to forget how powerful they can be. In addition to the cautions listed with each pose throughout the book, the general cautions below will make your restorative yoga practice safe and satisfying, and will maximize the benefits.

- The poses and programs presented are not intended to take the place of professional medical advice. If you have particular health concerns, for example, a back injury or abnormal blood pressure, show this book to your health care professional before beginning practice, and discuss how you can integrate the practice of restorative yoga into your health care regime.

- Pay special attention to the comfort of your neck and lower back. Specific information is given with the instructions for each pose.

- Do not practice inverted yoga poses if you have a hiatal hernia, retinal problems, glaucoma, migraine headaches, heart problems, neck problems, or an infection in your head.

- Women should not practice inverted poses or place weight on the abdomen during menstruation. Other special instructions for menstruation, pregnancy, and menopause are detailed in chapters 12, 13, and 14. Please review each chapter carefully before practice.

Be bold. If you're going to make an error, make a doozy, and don't be afraid to hit the ball.
—**Billie Jean King**

- Be careful about driving immediately after a restorative practice. You may feel very relaxed, so take transition time to make sure you are fully alert.

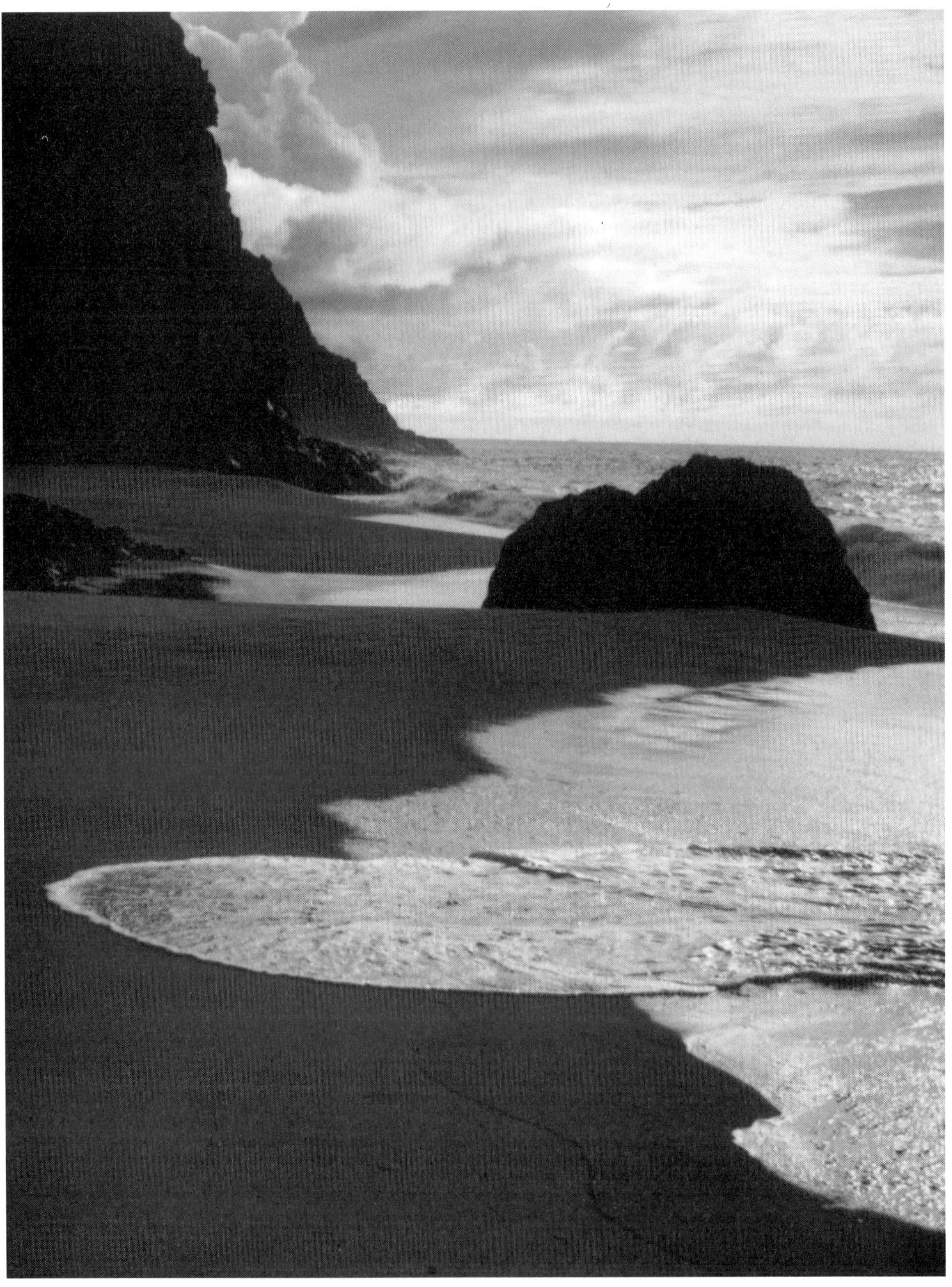

CHAPTER THREE

PROPS

Getting It Together

RESTORATIVE POSES are poses of being rather than doing. In practicing them, you are usually asked to lie down and support your head and limbs with props. While each restorative pose requires only a few props, a sequence of poses may use more.

To make things easier, I have organized the props by category. And for convenient visual reference, I have designed two charts (see end of chapter). The Props Chart (figure 3.1) describes each prop and its approximate dimensions. You can either purchase props from the providers listed in Resources in the appendix, or use the suggested alternatives to create props from things you might have around the house. The Blanket Chart (figure 3.2) shows you how to prepare blankets for practice. I have named each of the folds for easier reference throughout the book.

I cannot emphasize enough how important it is that you are comfortable when practicing. Key places to check for tension and holding are in your lower back, your abdomen, and your neck and jaw muscles. If you are uncomfortable, come out of the pose and rearrange your props. You may need to change the dimensions or placement of what you are using or try another prop. With some practice, you'll know exactly what you need and where to place it. Your attention to your comfort will be worth the effort.

Props You Lie Over

I believe that the physical is the geography of being.
—LOUISE NEVELSON

Blankets are the most important and versatile prop. You can spread a blanket on the floor for padding or insulation. You may also need a blanket to cover yourself if you feel cool. Blankets used for these two purposes can be of any type, including afghans, quilts, or even a mattress pad. However, when you use blankets as props, you need twin-size, firm, preferably wool blankets. If you are allergic to wool, use firm cotton blankets instead. Don't use blankets that are plush or thermal. Firm blankets give better support and are easier to fold into various shapes.

The standard-fold blanket is our basic blanket prop configuration. Fold your twin-size blanket in half three times, until it is approximately 21 x 28 inches. Starting with this shape, we add other folds to support the knees, neck, and head. Refer to the Blanket Chart (figure 3.2), which describes various folds. If you take a few moments to practice folding your blankets, you will enhance your practice significantly.

At least one large, firm bolster is used in many of the restorative poses. While three or more single-fold blankets can take the place of a bolster, if you own one bolster, you reduce the required number of blankets.

Yoga blocks are usually made of wood or foam, but you can substitute anything firm with the correct dimensions. If you are using a stack of books, tie them together so they do not slide apart. Sometimes the block bears a significant amount of body weight, so if you are improvising, use a material that will not collapse.

You can get nonskid mats from suppliers of props. I do not recommend using carpet pads that are rubbery or made up of foam particles; they are thin and shred easily. Use the mat to cover the floor where you practice; you can also roll it or fold it to take the place of a blanket. In a few cases, you use it so you do not slip in the pose.

For some poses I ask you to place a pillow under your heels or to lie on a folded towel to support your neck. A bed or sofa pillow works just fine. The ideal towel is a standard-size, thin cotton bath towel.

Props You Place on Your Body

Belts specifically designed for yoga are generally about 6 feet long and 2 inches wide and have a wide D-shaped buckle. An alternative belt should be wide and soft, so it does not cut into your skin.

A yoga sandbag is used to apply pressure to the body in a relatively small area. If you make your own sandbag, it should be supple and dense. Make sure the covering is strong and nonporous. Fill it with coarse well sand, not beach sand. If the sand is too fine, the bag will leak with use.

Iyengar maintains that if the head and face are relaxed, the body follows. Covering the eyes adds considerably to the depth of the relaxation. An eyebag is a small, rectangular cloth bag, usually made of silk or soft cotton, that is filled with uncooked rice, or flax seeds, or washable plastic beads, and is used to cover the eyes. The filling is loose enough that it moves easily in the bag and can be adjusted to lightly fill the eye sockets, giving gentle pressure to the eyes and the muscles around them. If you don't have an eyebag, you can use a soft cloth to shield your eyes from the light.

In each pose there should be repose.
—B.K.S. Iyengar

Another eye covering that many people find useful is an elastic bandage that is about 4 inches wide, the kind of bandage you use to wrap an injured ankle. They are available at most drug stores. It makes an ideal head wrap, especially in the case of headache or insomnia. Details about using this wrap are given in conjunction with specific poses.

For some poses, I suggest placing one or two rolled towels under your ankles or behind your knees to create more room in these joints. The ideal towel for this is a standard-size, thin, cotton bath towel.

Props You Rest On or Against

The common requirement for each of the props in this category is that they be sturdy enough to support your body weight.

The chair can be a metal folding chair, an armchair, or a wooden kitchen chair. For your safety, select one without rollers or casters.

Make sure the doorknob you use is securely assembled. A traditional round doorknob is easiest to work with. The door should be solidly attached to its hinges. A door with three hinges (usually an outside door) is stronger than one with two.

The table can be a dining table or desk. Make sure it will not slide if you lean against it.

Clear a wall space to use for your practice. If you don't have a space, you can use the back of a closed door, a large piece of furniture like an armoire or bookcase, or even the refrigerator.

FIGURE 3.1
Props Chart

Props You Lie Over

Prop	Qty.	Description	Dimensions	Alternatives
Blanket	3–7	firmly pressed or woven wool or cotton	62" x 80"	thick bath towels; quilts; rolled or folded nonskid mat; sofa cushions
Block	1	wood or recycled foam	4" x 6" x 9"	stack of hardcover books, tied together; telephone book
Bolster	1	cotton-filled cushion with round edges	9" x 9" x 27"	blankets; thick bath towels; couch cushions
Mat	1	nonskid	1/8" x 24" x 68"	nonslip floor
Pillow	1	from bed or sofa		folded towel or blanket
Towel	2	standard-size bath, thin cotton	2' x 3'	folded cloth

Props You Place On Your Body

Prop	Qty.	Description	Dimensions	Alternatives
Belt	1	cotton, with D-ring buckle	1.5" x 72"	wide bathrobe tie; 2 wide neckties tied together
Elastic Bandage	1	athletic-type wrap commonly found at pharmacy	4" x 48"	eyebag
Eyebag	1	8-oz. silk- or cotton-covered bag, filled with washable plastic beads, or uncooked rice, or flax seeds	1" x 4" x 8.5"	facecloth folded to measure 3" x 12"
Sandbag	1	10-lb. sand-filled bag covered with durable fabric	2" x 7" x 17"	package of rice, beans, or sugar

Props You Rest On Or Against

Prop	Qty.	Description	Dimensions	Alternatives
Chair	1	folding type preferred	standard	sturdy, wooden or metal chair, without rollers or casters
Door & Doorknob	1	3-hinge door with securely attached knob	standard	sturdy column or post
Table	1	sturdy	waist height x shoulder width	cover with nonskid mat and use folded blankets to achieve correct height
Wall	1	flat, bare (free of windows, decorations)	shoulder height x shoulder width	any clear, flat, solid, sturdy vertical surface

Figure 3.2
Blanket Chart

Standard-Fold
1" x 21" x 28"

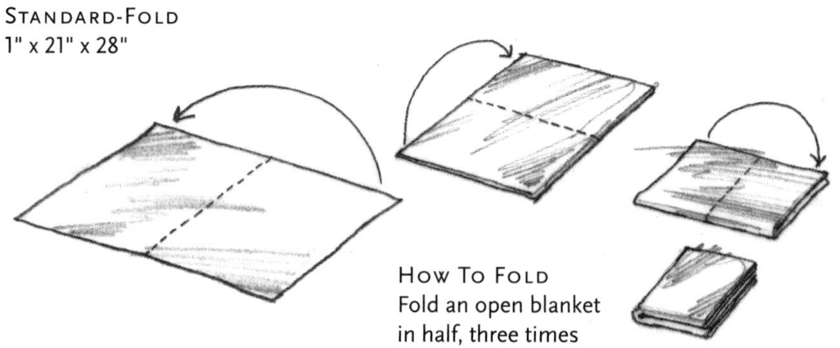

How To Fold
Fold an open blanket in half, three times

Single-Fold
2.5" x 10" x 28"

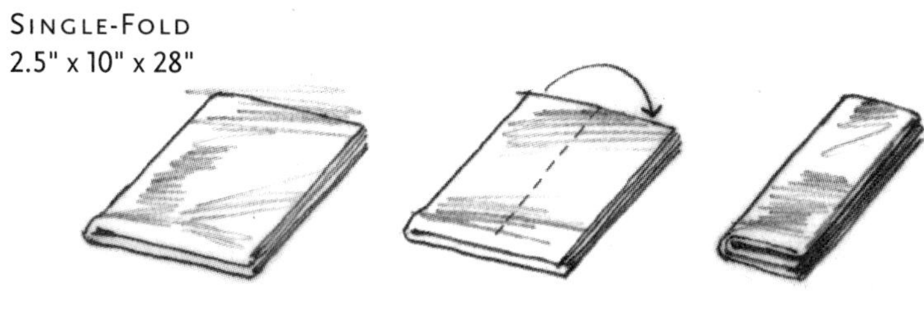

How To Fold
Standard-fold;
fold in half lengthwise

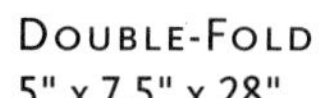
Double-Fold
5" x 7.5" x 28"

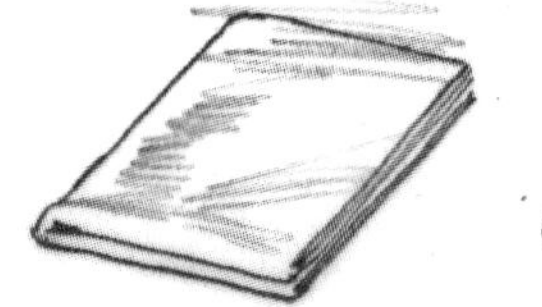
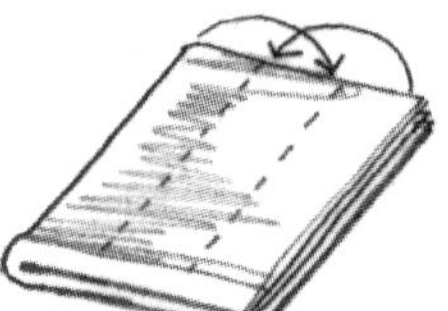
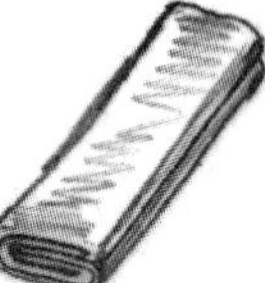

How To Fold
Standard-fold;
two folds lengthwise

Long-Roll
5" x 6" x 28"

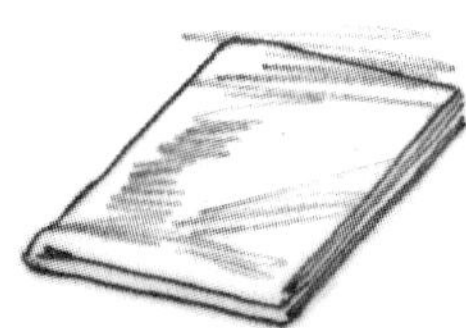

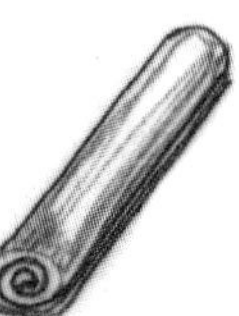

How To Fold
Standard-fold; start at long folded edge and roll blanket

CHAPTER FOUR

THE HEART OF PRACTICE

Basic Relaxation Pose

THE FOUNDATION of restorative yoga, Basic Relaxation Pose is the practice of deliberate stillness. Most of our lives are spent in movement. The fetus begins to move in the womb within the first few weeks. Our days are filled with high-tech conveniences that allow us to get more done, faster. Even during sleep we move about to find a more comfortable position. The yoga antidote is the simple act of lying down and being still.

What happens next? Outer stillness is just the beginning. By lying down, you quiet the gross movements of the body. This gives you entrance to a rich inner landscape. To your initial surprise, you discover that nothing is still. There is the rise and fall of the abdomen with the breath, the heart beating, the blood moving through the veins; gurgling sounds may come from the abdomen. And there is the mind, jumping from thought to thought, from past to future, resisting stillness.

Why spend time in Basic Relaxation Pose if everything is always moving? Is relaxation even possible? It is. As the props relieve your muscles and bones of their roles of support and action, your nervous system sends and receives fewer messages and becomes quieter. Layers of tension melt away as you learn to be present to what is happening in the body and mind in each moment.

In short, Basic Relaxation Pose and the other restorative poses cultivate the habit of attention. You learn to identify how and where you hold tension and consciously release it. You discover a clear space from which to make life choices. Through restorative poses, you come into harmony with your body's natural rhythms. Living by these rhythms is the key to good health.

The Centering Breath

Like other relaxation techniques, Basic Relaxation Pose places the body in a comfortable position, with gentle attention directed toward the breath. One way to include the breath in practice is a simple exercise called the Centering Breath. It is subtle practice with many benefits, including increased respiratory capacity and lowered blood pressure. The Centering Breath is recommended for many supine poses throughout this book. You will be referred back to these instructions and to the Being There section on page 26.

Know thy self.
—PLATO

To practice:

1. Take a long, slow, gentle inhalation through your nose.
2. Follow the inhalation with a long, slow, gentle exhalation through your nose.
3. Take several normal cycles of breath through your nose until you feel refreshed.
4. Repeat steps 1, 2, and 3 for up to 10 rounds.

Never strain or force the breath. The success of the Centering Breath is not measured by how much air you can take in or let out. So go slowly, gently, and be present with the process. If you feel fatigued, anxious, or light-headed during practice, it is an indication that you have practiced long enough. Let your breathing return to normal, and in the future, take longer breaks of normal breathing between each round of long inhalation and long exhalation. Do not practice the Centering Breath if you have a fever, a bad cold, sinusitis, or more serious respiratory diseases, such as pneumonia.

Remember, each breath is another sign that life is moving through you; enjoy it.

Basic Relaxation Pose

The less time you think you have for spending a few minutes a day in Basic Relaxation Pose, the more you need to do it. If you do nothing else for your health every day, make time for this pose. Practice it, for example, in an afternoon break at work, when you first come home from work, after an exercise session, or whenever you feel depleted, exhausted, or stressed.

Prop

- standard-fold blanket

Optional Props

- eyebag
- long-roll blanket
- pillow
- extra blanket for warmth
- clock or timer

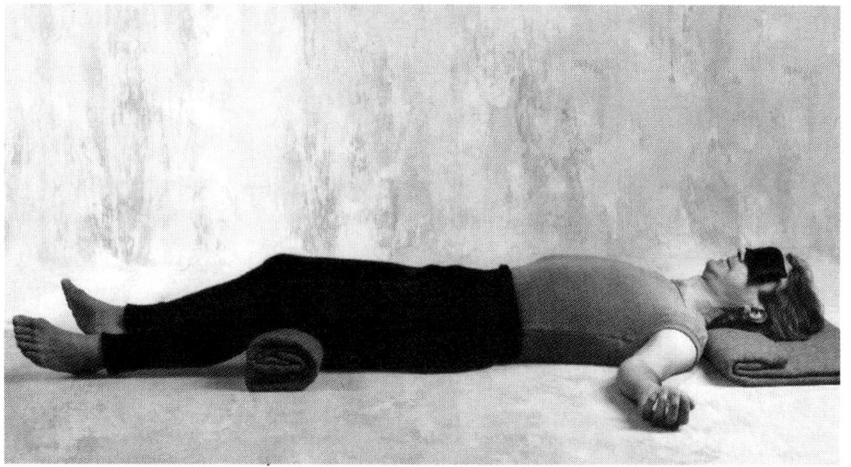

FIGURE 4.1
Basic Relaxation Pose

You can create several variations of Basic Relaxation Pose by using different props. Once you have become familiar with the Basic Relaxation Pose presented in this chapter, try the variations in other chapters. Throughout the book, you will be referred back to this complete description of Basic Relaxation Pose. Once you are more familiar with the pose, you may not need to read the full instructions each time.

Setting Up. You will be lying on your back with your arms out to the sides and your legs comfortably apart. Give yourself enough floor space to spread out comfortably. Before you lie down, position a standard-fold blanket for your head and neck to rest on.

> Man must touch the spiritual at some point.
> —B.K.S. IYENGAR

Begin by sitting on the floor. If you have difficulty getting down to and up from the floor, see chapter 2 for helpful suggestions. If you have a tendency to get cold, cover your legs with an unfolded blanket. Now turn to one side, and lean on your elbow and forearm as you slide onto your side. Then roll onto your back. Coming into the pose in this way is less stressful on your back than leaning back into a reclining position.

Roll the long edge of your standard-fold blanket slightly to support

There is nothing stronger in the world than tenderness.
—HAN SUYIN

the gentle curve of the neck. Adjust the prop placement so your neck is comfortable. Your chin should be slightly lower than your forehead. This position quiets the frontal lobes of the brain. If you are using an extra blanket for warmth, now is the time to pull it up to cover your torso and arms. Cover your eyes with an eyebag.

Many people can practice this pose lying flat on the floor. But if you have tension or pain in your abdomen or lower back, place a long-roll blanket under the backs of your knees before you lie down. Make sure that your legs are relaxed and the knees supported by the long-roll blanket. If your heels do not touch the floor, place a folded blanket or pillow under them. If your lower back discomfort persists, come out of the pose by following the instructions under Coming Back (below), and try practicing Side-Lying Relaxation Pose (see chapter 13). Resume your practice of Basic Relaxation Pose when you feel ready.

Once you have established yourself, observe the position of your body. Your arms and legs should be equidistant from an imaginary line drawn from the tip of your nose to exactly midway between the feet. Most people practice with the palms turned upward, but if this is not comfortable, turn them down and let the elbows relax. The most important thing is that you feel completely at ease and supported by the props and the floor. If you need to sit up to adjust props and lie down again, follow the instructions for Coming Back and Setting Up.

Being There. Swallow and relax your lower jaw. Soften your upper eyelids and look down toward the lower lids as you close your eyes. Let your cheeks feel hollow and loose beneath the cheekbones. Release the root of your tongue. Your fingers will curl naturally as your hands relax. Let your legs roll outward. Allow the entire back of your body to feel at ease and in complete contact with the floor and the props.

Your arms and legs will feel longer and longer, as well as heavier. Feel the large muscles of the legs, buttocks, and trunk drop away from the bones. Now feel the smaller muscles of your arms, neck, and head as they seem to move away from the bones. Let the bones themselves feel heavy and the skin loose, all over your body. Notice that the abdominal organs seem to nestle gently back into your body. Savor the silence.

The Centering Breath. As you continue to rest, notice when you begin to feel lighter. This is a signal that your body has relaxed and that you can begin the Centering Breath: a long inhalation followed by a long exhalation, followed by several cycles of normal breathing.

Begin by slowly inviting the inhalation to move more deeply into your body. Do this by lifting your ribs slightly and spreading your lungs.

Let the air come to you. As you inhale, imagine that the breath breathes you. Follow the inhalation with a soft focus on the exhalation. Feel your diaphragm, lungs, ribs, and muscles of respiration contracting to press the breath out in a steady and focused stream. When your exhalation is finished, breathe several normal cycles of inhalation and exhalation.

Then inhale slowly and deeply once again. At the fullness of inhalation, pause slightly before melting the inhalation into an equally long and steady exhalation. The inhalation is the receptive part of the breath; the exhalation is the active part. Once again, take several normal cycles of breath.

Once you have established the rhythm of the long breaths, pay particular attention to the quality of these breaths. What is their texture? Is the beginning of inhalation as soft as the end of inhalation? Is the end of exhalation as smooth as the beginning? With each cycle, allow your breath to become more and more refined, like the texture of fine silk.

Remember, never force the breath. If at any time you feel even slightly agitated or out of breath, simply return to normal breathing. Once you feel calm, resume the cycle of long, slow inhalation and exhalation, followed by several normal breaths.

Repeat the Centering Breath for up to 10 rounds. Be sure to leave some time for normal breathing before coming out of the pose.

Coming Back. Remain in Basic Relaxation Pose for 5 to 20 minutes. To come out of the pose, bend one knee and roll onto your side. Let the eyebag fall off by itself. Gradually open your eyes. Rest in this position for a few breaths. To sit up, press the floor with the elbow of your lower arm and the palm of the hand of your upper arm. Sit quietly for several breaths before standing up and resuming your normal activities.

We are free to be at peace with ourselves and others, and also with nature.
—THOMAS MERTON

Benefits. Basic Relaxation Pose lowers blood pressure and heart rate, releases muscular tension, reduces fatigue, improves sleep, enhances immune response, and helps to manage chronic pain.

Caution

- If you are more than three months pregnant, practice Side-Lying Relaxation Pose (see chapter 13).

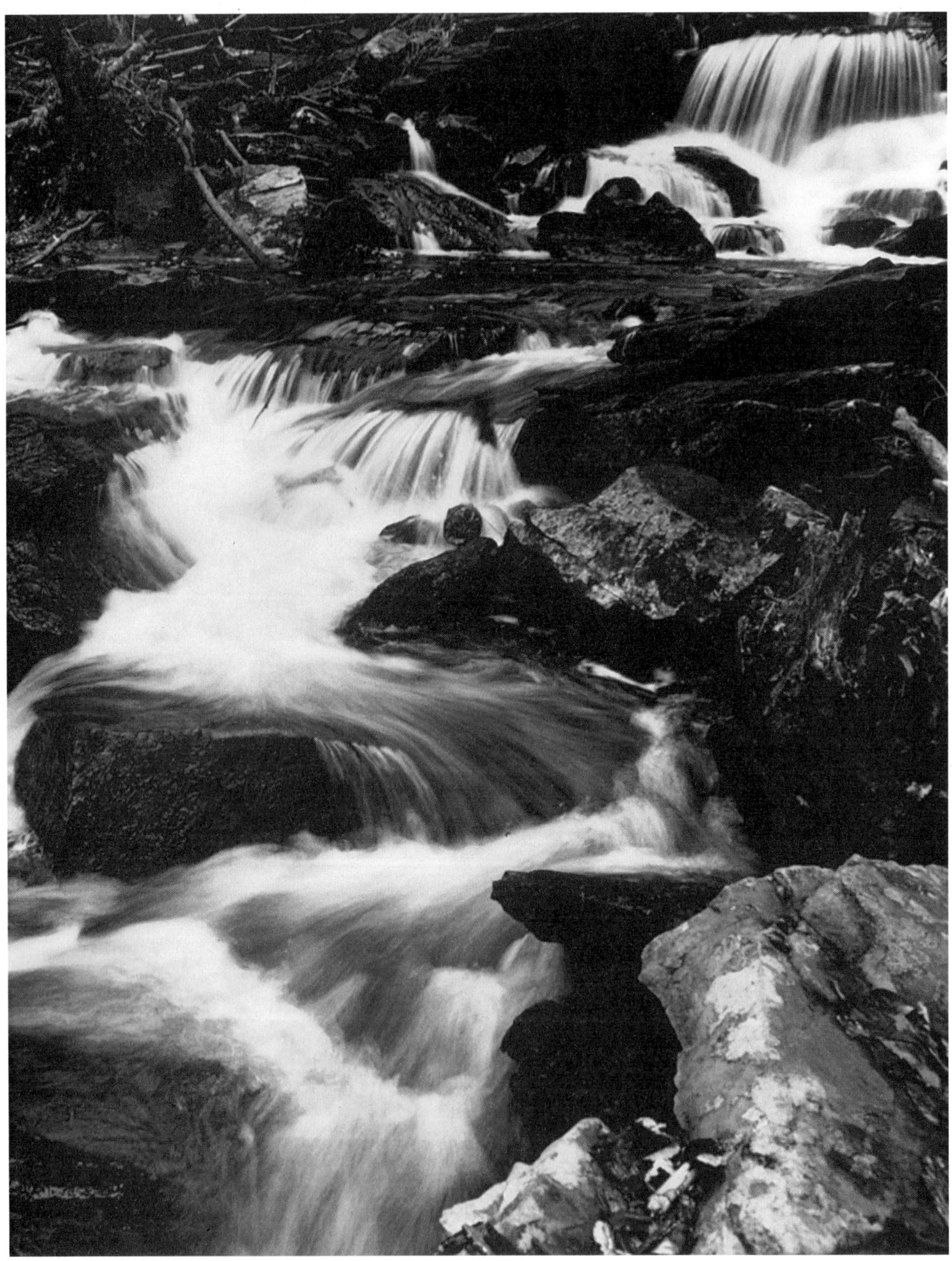

CHAPTER FIVE

RELAX AND RENEW

A General Restorative Practice

THERE IS NOTHING mysterious about practicing restorative poses: you gather the props you need, set yourself up in a pleasant space, then settle in and relax. Unlike other exercise programs, restorative poses place minimal metabolic demand on you. They add to your energy rather than subtract from it. During these periods of deep relaxation, you will be healed and nurtured from within.

I did restorative poses only occasionally in the early years of my yoga practice. Then a member of my extended family died, and I did not feel inspired to practice my usual yoga routine. In response to my grief, I decided to practice only restorative poses and did so almost every day for a year. It was practicing these poses, I believe, that helped me through this painful period. They allowed me to accept my grief and recover from the emotional drain and fatigue. In fact, it was my direct experience of the profound effects of restorative poses during that year that inspired me to write this book.

The Relax and Renew Series

> If anything is sacred,
> the human body is sacred.
> —Walt Whitman

This chapter presents a general restorative series, which I call Relax and Renew. While Basic Relaxation Pose is beneficial practiced by itself, it is even more so when practiced in a well-rounded sequence that moves the spine in all directions and stimulates and refreshes the abdominal organs.

The Relax and Renew series begins with a gentle back bend and progresses into deeper ones. Next is an inversion, or upside down pose, which reduces fatigue but is still somewhat stimulating on the scale of restorative poses. A twist follows to relieve any residual back tension from the back-bending movements. The series concludes with supported forward bends, which are cooling and introspective and will help you finish your practice in a quiet state, preparing you for Basic Relaxation Pose at the end.

The Relax and Renew series takes from 60 to 90 minutes. This timing does not include setting up, transition time from pose to pose, or staying longer in the poses. Do what you can, and always end with at least a 5-minute Basic Relaxation Pose. Naturally your first few experiences will take more time as you refine your use of the suggested props.

Many poses in this sequence can be practiced individually, especially Basic Relaxation Pose. Elevated Legs-Up-the-Wall Pose is a good refresher by itself, recommended for those with mild hypertension that is currently being controlled with medication. In fact, it can help to lower blood pressure. If your back and legs hurt, practice Supported Crossed-Legs Pose for 3 to 5 minutes as an isolated stress reducer. For busy days, you can also refer to the shorter routines in chapter 6. As you become more familiar with the practice, you will develop an understanding for what you need each day.

Take the time to familiarize yourself with the information in this chapter. Determine the props you will need. Gather them into your practice space so they are close at hand and you can move easily from one pose to the next. You may want to sit quietly for a few minutes before beginning just to slow down a little. For tips on how to sit comfortably, see chapter 17. You can also begin the Relax and Renew series with Basic Relaxation Pose, as described here or in chapter 4, and then move on to the following poses.

Simple Supported Back Bend

Many of us sit at work for much of the day with the spine rounded and the arms forward of the torso. As a result, tension accumulates in the muscles of the upper back and shoulders. In response, most of us have the urge to stretch our arms upward and bend backward. That is just what this pose helps us to do, but in a supported way.

Props

- bolster
- long-roll blanket

Optional Props

- eyebag
- block
- double-fold blanket
- extra blanket for warmth
- clock or timer

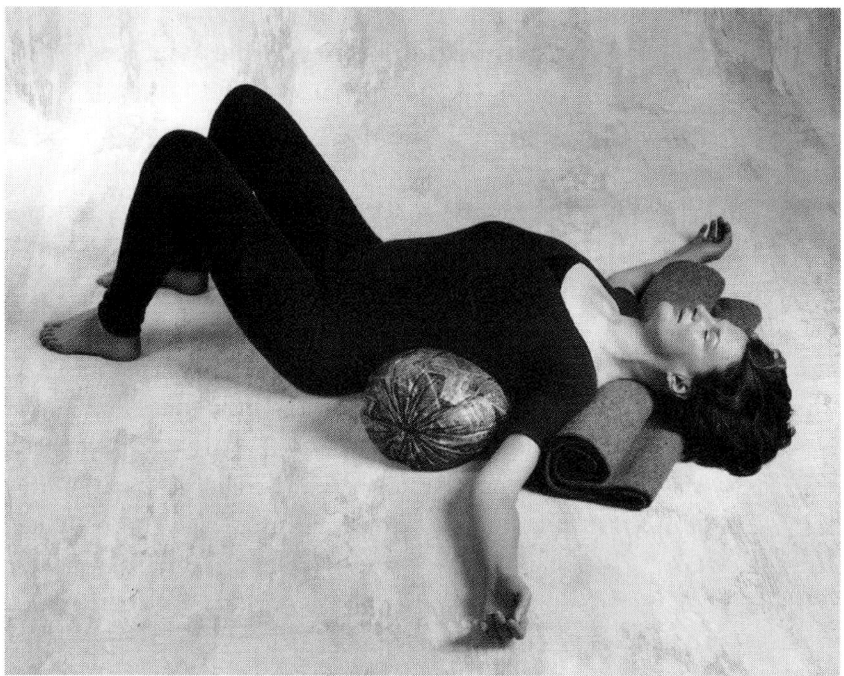

FIGURE 5.1
Simple Supported Back Bend

Setting Up. To begin, sit on the floor in front of the long side of your bolster, knees bent and feet resting on the floor, with a long-roll blanket by your side. Move slowly and with caution. If lying back causes discomfort in your lower back, begin by lying on your side over the bolster and then turning onto your back. If you can lie back, place your elbows on the bolster. Then use one hand to support your neck as you take your head back. Now lie over the bolster so that your mid back is supported by it and your shoulders rest comfortably on the floor.

The length of your torso will affect your comfort in this pose. Some short people have long torsos; some tall people have short ones. If you are long from shoulders to hips, place a double-fold blanket on the bolster to increase the height. This modification will allow you to rest lightly on your shoulders without crunching your neck against the floor. If

We are always getting ready to live but never living.
—Ralph Waldo Emerson

you are short from the shoulders to hips, you may be more comfortable with less height. If you use props that are too high for you, your head will hang without support.

Be careful not to put too much weight on your cervical spine (neck). Place the long-roll blanket under your shoulders. If it's too high, unroll it until you are comfortable. This support helps to maintain the natural curve of the neck and allows your throat to open and relax. Keep your knees bent throughout the pose to protect your back and relax the abdomen. If you find it more comfortable, let the knees rest against each other. Rest your arms on the floor, either above your head or out to the side, whichever is more pleasant. Breathe naturally.

Stay in the pose for 30 seconds to determine how you feel. If you experience any discomfort in your lower back, slightly move off the bolster in the direction of your head. If this fails to relieve it, slightly move off the bolster toward your feet or place your feet on a folded blanket. Make sure that your chest is open and your ribs lift away from the abdominal organs.

If none of these adjustments make the pose feel good, roll carefully to one side and sit up. The following adjustment usually does the trick: reduce the degree of the arch. Place the short side of a block against the front of the long side of the bolster. Sit on the block and use the support of your hands on the floor to lie back. Continue to use the roll under your shoulders to enhance your comfort and to protect your neck. Your tailbone and part of your buttocks should be supported by the block. There should be some arch in your back, especially at the level of your shoulder blades. Close your eyes. Place the eyebag over them.

Being There. Breathe slowly and evenly. Feel held by the props. Your arms are wide open and free. With each inhalation, your front body opens; with each exhalation, your belly and organs soften and your mind quiets. As you gradually relax, allow your back to sink into the props. Imagine you are lying in a beautiful and safe space. Open to this place, and receive the beauty and wholeness of this moment.

Coming Back. Practice Simple Supported Back Bend for 1 minute, gradually increasing your time in the pose. To come out, remove the eyebag. Push with your feet and slide toward your head. Rest for a few breaths with your lower back flat on the floor and your legs supported by the bolster. Then roll to the side and sit up slowly.

Benefits. Simple Supported Back Bend is an antidote to our habitual posture of rounding forward. The front of the body is energized, and the abdominal organs are stimulated. This back bend will leave you feeling refreshed.

Cautions

Do not practice this pose:

- if you experience pain in your lower back in the pose. Do allow for the sensation of stretch, which might feel unusual, especially if you have been protecting your lower back.
- if you have spondylolisthesis, spondylolysis, or diagnosed disc disease.
- if you are more than three months pregnant. Practice the restorative series in chapter 13 instead.
- during menstruation. Practice the restorative series in chapter 12 instead.

Supported Bound-Angle Pose

Supported Bound-Angle Pose is one of the most important in the restorative series. Physically it opens the chest, abdomen, and pelvis. These areas are often restricted by the ways we stand and sit, the shape of our chairs, and even the fit of our clothes. Psychologically it allows for a deep opening with safety and support. As the chest opens, the arms and legs are cradled by the props.

In *The Yoga Sutras,* the Indian sage Patanjali writes about *hiranyagarbha,*

Props

- bolster
- 4 long-roll blankets
- double-fold blanket
- belt or sandbag

Optional Props

- single-fold blanket
- eyebag
- extra blanket for warmth
- clock or timer

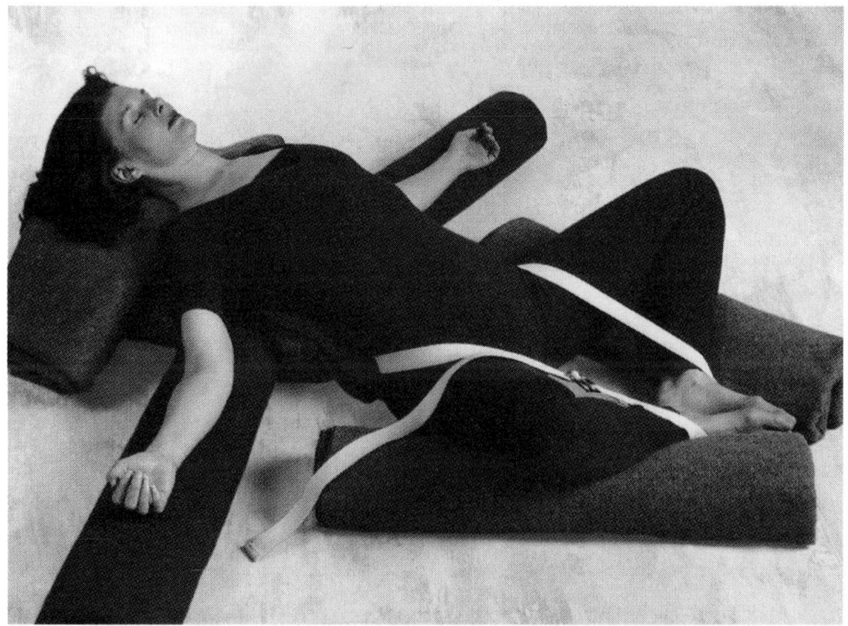

FIGURE 5.2
Supported Bound-Angle Pose

Practice is absolutely necessary.
—SWAMI VIVEKANANDA

a Sanskrit word that means "the great golden womb of the universe."[1] Patanjali teaches that the entire universe is held within this golden womb. As we practice Supported Bound-Angle Pose, we are reminded of this primordial place of complete rest and ultimate protection. While lying in this pose, I have experienced being held within this force. This experience is profoundly comforting and leaves me with a feeling of equanimity and well-being.

One of the most relaxing of all restorative poses, Supported Bound-Angle Pose requires some patience to set up. but it is well worth the effort. You rest on supports for your back, neck, and head, and then you put the bottoms of your feet together and let your knees fall out to the side. The position of the legs is the bound angle. The feet are held together by the angle of the bent knees. Extra support goes under your forearms and outer thighs to make the pose even more comfortable.

Setting Up. Sit in front of the short end of your bolster, with it touching your tailbone. Bend your knees and place your feet on the floor. Use your arms for support as you gently lie down. The bolster should support you from your sacrum to your head. If you feel any discomfort in your lower back, adjust the height of the support. You can increase the height of the bolster by adding a single-fold blanket; you can decrease the height by practicing with the single-fold blanket instead of a bolster.

Once you are comfortable, place a double-fold blanket under your neck and head. Make sure that your entire neck is adequately supported by the prop. Your head should not be too high or low. Your forehead should be higher than your chin, your chin higher than your breastbone, and your breastbone higher than your pubic bone. Once positioned, your torso should be at a 45-degree angle to the floor.

Place the soles of your feet together, and let your knees fall to the sides. Place a long-roll blanket under each outer thigh. *Use the long-roll blankets even if you are supple and open easily in this direction.* These blankets should completely support the weight of your legs so you experience no traction in the sacral ligaments, which are extremely vulnerable in this position. Make sure that the knees are at equal heights from the floor. Remember, the point of the pose is not to stretch the inner thighs but to relax the abdomen and open the chest. Once you have determined the right prop configuration for you, roll to one side and use your arms to help you come to a sitting position.

As you relax, your feet may slide away from you. A belt or sandbag will hold your feet in position so your legs can relax. Fasten your belt into a loop long enough to accommodate the distance from your hips to your feet when lying down. Bring the belt over your head and position it around your hips. With the soles of your feet together, wrap the free side of the loop around your feet. Be careful to place the buckle where it will not press against your skin. The belt should not be too tight. To help you secure the belt once you lie down, position the loose end pointing toward your hand. If you have a sandbag, you can use it instead of a belt. Place it across your feet to hold them in place.

Position 2 more long-roll blankets to support your forearms, and lie down again. Make sure that each forearm is positioned in the middle of its long-roll blanket, parallel with the edges of the blanket. This added support will give you the feeling of floating and can relieve any stretch on the nerves of the neck and arms, particularly important if you have neck problems. This support also helps to relax the shoulders. Place an eyebag over your eyes.

Posture should be steady and comfortable.

—Yoga Sutras of Patanjali, II:46

Being There. Supported Bound-Angle Pose provides an excellent opportunity to practice the Centering Breath: a slow, gentle inhalation, followed by a slow, gentle exhalation, followed by several normal cycles of breath, until you feel refreshed and ready to begin the Centering Breath again. (See pages 24 and 26 for complete instructions.) Repeat this process for up to 10 breaths. Be sure to leave some time for normal breathing before coming out of the pose.

Coming Back. Practice Supported Bound-Angle Pose for 10 to 15 minutes. Some people prefer to make this pose the focus of their restorative practice and remain as long as 30 minutes. After relaxing so deeply, let the outside world come slowly into your awareness. Take in the sounds around you; pay attention to the sensations of your body.

When you feel ready, remove the eyebag and slowly open your eyes. To come up, press down with your arms and sit up slowly. Undo the belt or remove the sandbag from your feet. Slowly stretch your legs out in front of you to release any tension in the knees. Carefully move to the next pose or on to the rest of your day.

Benefits. Supported Bound-Angle Pose benefits those with high blood pressure and breathing problems. It is also helpful for women during the menstrual period (see chapter 12) and during menopause (see chapter 14).

Cautions

- If you have disc disease in your lower back or chronic sacroiliac dysfunction, lower the height of the props, still keeping your head higher than your chest and your chest higher than your pelvis.

- If you have a pinched nerve or disc disease in your neck, carefully support your head and neck. Experiment with the height and position of your props so you can practice symptom-free. For example, tingling down the arms may indicate that you are straining your neck.
- If you have a knee injury, bending it for long periods of time can be uncomfortable. Practice this pose for short periods at first. Be sure to give adequate support to the outsides of your thighs to protect your knees.
- If you feel stiff after coming out of the pose and moving around for the first few minutes, practice for less time the next time. Stiffness can come from overstretching the ligaments of your pelvis by practicing the pose for too long.

Do not practice this pose:

- if you have spondylolisthesis or spondylolysis.
- if you experience discomfort in your neck, lower back, or knees even after experimenting with prop height and placement.

Mountain Brook Pose

Props

- bolster
- 2 single-fold blankets
- long-roll blanket

Optional Props

- standard-fold blanket
- eyebag
- extra blanket for warmth
- clock or timer
- facecloth

In Mountain Brook Pose, your body is gently draped in a wavelike pattern over the props, like water flowing over the stones in a mountain

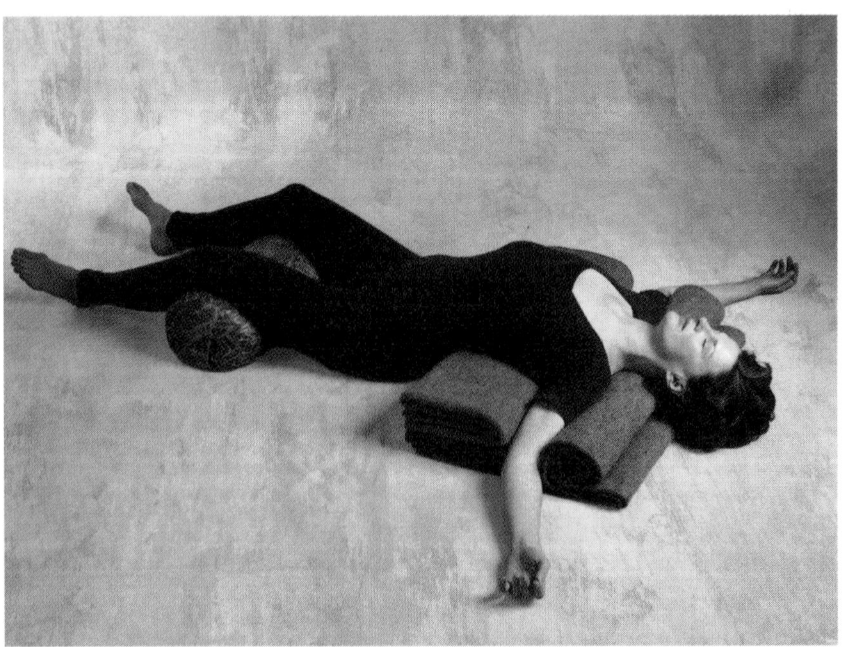

FIGURE 5.3
Mountain Brook Pose

brook. While opening your chest, as in Simple Supported Back Bend, Mountain Brook Pose adds two supports: one under your knees and the other behind your neck. With the help of the props, this pose allows for an opening in three areas we generally protect: the throat, the heart, and the belly.

Setting Up. Sit in front of the long side of 2 stacked single-fold blankets. Lie over them to determine if the height and placement feel right. For most people, the center line of the blanket is best placed just below the shoulder blades. If you feel overarched, use only 1 single-fold blanket or 1 standard-fold blanket with a single-fold blanket. As always, take the time necessary to find the right height of your props. Now roll to one side and slowly sit up.

Peace within makes beauty without.
—ENGLISH PROVERB

Place the bolster under your knees, and position the long-roll blanket to support your neck. Lie back with these three props in place.

Scan your body to make sure you are comfortable. The arch of your neck should be completely supported. Your head tilts gently backward, and your throat is open and relaxed. The bolster under your knees protects your lower back. Your arms are placed out to the side at approximately 90 degrees, but whatever is comfortable is fine.

If you feel any discomfort, roll to one side and slowly sit up. Lower the height of the middle blankets or increase the height of the prop under your knees, and lie back again. I cannot emphasize often enough that when this pose is properly set up, your neck should be completely relaxed. Close your eyes and place an eyebag over them.

Note: This restorative pose is unique because it is done with the head hanging back, with the cervical spine (neck) in extension, or back bending. When you are setting up, make sure your head is back so the throat is open, like your chest and belly. You will likely enjoy a small, rolled facecloth under the lowest part of your neck to support the cervical spine. Do not support the middle of the neck, as this will only serve to increase the curve, not support it. If you are uncomfortable after trying to support your neck, perhaps skip this pose. Do skip this pose if you have concerns about placing your cervical spine in extension.

Being There. Breathe normally. Let go of all the parts of your body you use to speak, beginning with the muscles behind your ears, down through the jaw, and all the way to your chin. Allow your lips to part slightly. Let your tongue rest easily in your mouth, and let your cheeks feel as though they are hollow and hanging from the cheekbones. Swallow to relax any tension in your throat. Give up any unspoken words.

As you continue to breathe and feel the support of the props, gently

Health is not a condition of matter, but of mind.
—Mary Baker Eddy

bring your attention to your heart. Receive whatever feelings arise from your heart. Some students tell me that this pose brings up feelings of sadness; others experience oceanic feelings of peace. Whatever arises, remain present.

And now to the belly, a more friendly name for the abdomen. Anatomically this area begins at the diaphragm, located at the base of the breastbone, and ends at the lower pelvis. With each exhalation, allow your belly to drop toward your spine. Imagine that your body is softening and spreading. As you continue to relax, you will feel more spacious and loose. Breathe normally, enjoying the freedom you feel in your throat, heart, and belly.

Coming Back. Practice Mountain Brook Pose for 5 minutes. If you are very comfortable or are an experienced yoga student, stay for as long as 15 minutes. If you have a stiff back, start with only a few minutes and gradually increase your time in the pose. To come out, remove the eyebag and use your hands to gently lift your head. Then use your hands to help you slide off the props toward your head. Let your legs rest on the bolster. Lie on the floor for a few minutes before rolling to one side and getting up.

Benefits. Mountain Brook Pose counteracts the slumped sitting posture that so many of our daily activities reinforce. In addition, it opens the chest to help you breathe more fully. The pose also improves digestion, reduces fatigue, and can lift your mood if you feel down.

Cautions

- If your back feels too stretched or stiff after the first few times, try this the next time: Before coming out of the pose, bring your legs to your chest one at a time as you exhale. Then roll to the side and sit up.

Do not practice this pose:

- if you have spondylolisthesis, spondylolysis, or disc disease.
- if you are more than three months pregnant.

When experiencing is steady, the breath will gradually become slow, long, and deep.
—Charlotte Joko Beck

Supported Bridge Pose

An inverted pose, Supported Bridge Pose gives us an experience of what Iyengar calls "negative brain." Here he does not mean negative as bad, but as cool, slow, and introspective. This restorative yoga pose is an antidote for living in an age that manipulates our brains and nervous systems into being hot, fast, and extroverted.

Props

- 2 bolsters

Optional Props

- 2 or more single-fold blankets
- eyebag
- towel
- extra blanket for warmth
- clock or timer

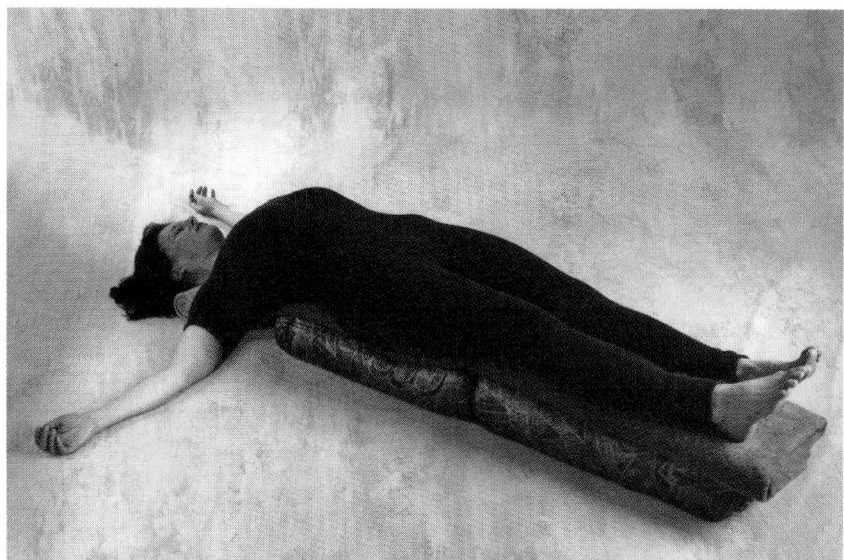

FIGURE 5.4
Supported Bridge Pose

Setting Up. Place the bolsters end-to-end to accommodate the length of your body. The height of the props depends on the length of your torso and the flexibility of your upper back. If your back is stiff, you can begin by using single-fold blankets and gradually increase the height. Most people find that props measuring 6 to 12 inches in height work well. If you are tall, try 2 bolsters with 2 or more single-fold blankets on top to create additional height. Make sure that the height of the props is even throughout their length.

Sit down, straddling the bolsters, and move slightly nearer to the end behind you. Use the support of your arms to help you lie down. Carefully slide off the end toward your head so your shoulders touch the floor and you face the ceiling. If you feel any discomfort in your lower back, bend your knees and place your feet either on top of the bolster or on the floor on either side.

To preserve the natural curve of your neck, be careful not to jam your chin into your chest. To counteract this tendency, use a rolled towel to support the vertebra (C7) located at the base of your neck, near the shoulders. Use a standard bath towel, the thinner the better. Fold the

Too many people, too many demands, too much to do; competent, busy, hurrying people—it just isn't living at all.
—ANNE MORROW LINDBERGH

towel in half longways, and then fold one end over about 6 to 8 inches. Starting at the fold, roll the towel and place it at the base of your neck, parallel to your shoulders. Do not support the middle of the neck where the curve is the greatest. Experiment with the size of the roll so you are comfortable. You can always reduce the size of the roll and let the unrolled part spread under your head.

Place an eyebag over your forehead or your eyes; place your arms out to the side at a comfortable angle.

Being There. Begin by making sure that you are comfortable. Gently bring your attention to your breathing. Feel the lateral movement of your lungs and ribs with each inhalation and exhalation. To enhance your relaxation, let your eyeballs turn downward. Let the energy of thought draw inward, as the energy of the body opens and expands.

Coming Back. Practice Supported Bridge Pose as long as you are comfortable, up to 15 minutes. To come out, remove the eyebag and slide off the bolsters in the direction of your head. Rest your lower legs on the bolster, with your back on the floor. Stay for a few minutes, and then roll to one side. Press down with your hands and sit up slowly.

Benefits. Supported Bridge Pose drains fluid from the legs after long periods of standing, thus reducing fatigue. Athletes find it beneficial after a long run to help reduce soreness in the leg and hip muscles. This pose also helps alleviate headaches (see chapter 8) or mental agitation, which are often the symptoms of overwork.

Cautions

- This pose is not recommended for those who should avoid inversions: individuals with hiatal hernias, eye pressure, retinal problems, heart problems, or neck problems, and menstruating women. If you have any concerns about practicing inverted poses, consult your health care professional.

Do not practice this pose:

- if you have spondylolisthesis or spondylolysis.
- after the first three months of pregnancy.
- if you have a respiratory or sinus infection.
- if you have indigestion.
- if you are recovering from whiplash or have any questions about the suitability of the pose for your neck.

Elevated Legs-Up-the-Wall Pose

Elevated Legs-Up-the-Wall Pose is another gentle inversion. The pelvis and torso are supported in a gentle back bend, while the wall supports the legs. With the help of gravity, the shape of the pose creates a waterfall, as the fluid in the legs cascades down, pools in the lagoon created by the shape of the belly, and then spills over into the chest.

I find Elevated Legs-Up-the-Wall Pose one of the most useful in the Relax and Renew series. It simultaneously revives the legs and relieves the back. I began to practice it when my children were young. We would line up in the hallway, all with legs up the wall, and I would read them a story aloud. Even the children found the pose relaxing.

Props

- bolster
- single-fold blanket

Optional Props

- eyebag
- double-fold blanket
- 1 or more single-fold blankets
- standard-fold blanket
- towel
- extra blanket for warmth
- clock or timer

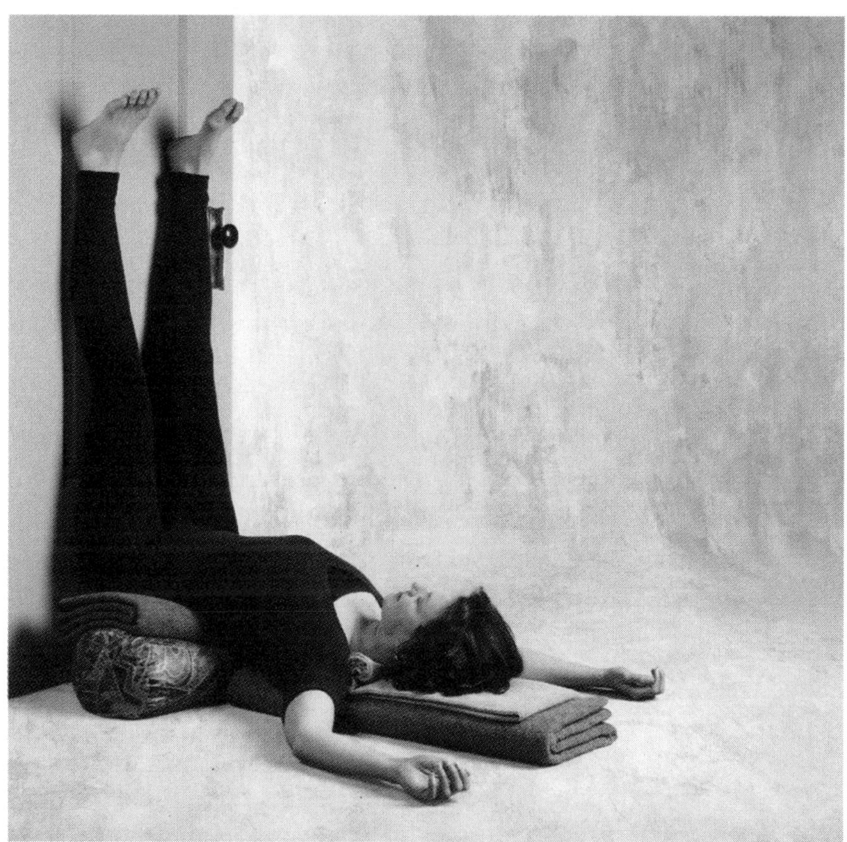

FIGURE 5.5
Elevated Legs-Up-the-Wall Pose

Setting Up. Place the long side of the bolster parallel to the wall, leaving about 6 to 10 inches between the wall and the bolster. Place a single-fold blanket on the floor at a 90-degree angle to the middle of the long side of the bolster.

Sit on one end of the bolster, with the length of the bolster behind you and one shoulder near the wall. Roll back and simultaneously swing your legs up the wall. This may take some practice to get right. People are usually are too close or too far from the wall the first time; do not be discouraged. Practice this part a few times until you feel you can do it smoothly and easily. If you still have trouble getting up, try the movement without the bolster so you learn the proper relationship to the wall. A common limitation in getting the legs up the wall is tightness in the backs of the legs. If you have this tightness, simply move the props farther from the wall and try again.

> The other side of anger, if we experience its emptiness and go through it, is compassion.
> —Charlotte Joko Beck

Once in position, your legs are almost vertical and your torso is in a half-dome shape. Remember, this is a relaxing pose, not a stretching one. You will not be able to relax if the backs of your legs are too stretched. In this case, you may need to readjust the props so they are farther from the wall.

Make sure your lower back is supported. Most people feel best when the ribs closest to the waist are supported by the bolster. If you are uncomfortable on the bolster, experiment with using blankets. If you need a narrow support, try a double-fold blanket on top of a single-fold blanket; if you need a wider support, 2 or 3 single-fold blankets may be your answer.

The height of the props is also very individual. You will not enjoy the pose if the props are too high or too low. If you have a long, flexible torso, you may need a standard-fold blanket or single-fold blanket on top of your bolster for extra height.

To preserve the natural curve of your neck, be careful not to jam your chin into your chest. To counteract this tendency, use a rolled towel to support the vertebra (C7) located at the base of your neck, near the shoulders. Use a standard bath towel, the thinner the better. Fold the towel in half lengthwise, and then fold one end over about 6 to 8 inches. Starting at the fold, roll the towel and place it at the base of your neck and parallel to your shoulders. Do not support the middle of the neck where the curve is the greatest. Experiment with the size of the roll so you are comfortable. You can always reduce the size of the roll and let the unrolled part spread under your head.

Let your arms rest on the floor, either at your sides or overhead. If your arms are overhead, you can support them on another bolster or blanket. Place the eyebag over your eyes.

Being There. Let yourself be supported by the bolster and the floor. Forget the outside world for a few minutes; allow yourself the important task of doing nothing. Take slow and steady breaths. Because your chest is supported in an open position, as in Supported Bridge Pose, you may experience a sense of release. Enjoy the sensation of fatigue draining from your legs, your back and shoulders opening, and your mind quieting.

Coming Back. Practice Elevated Legs-Up-the-Wall Pose for up to 15 minutes. To come out, remove the eyebag and bend your knees. Press your feet on the wall and lift your pelvis slightly. Push the bolster toward the wall with your hands, and slide your body away from the wall by pressing with your feet. Lie on the floor for a few moments, with your lower legs supported by the bolster. Roll to the side and get up slowly.

The body is my altar, and the postures are the prayers.
—**B.K.S. Iyengar**

Benefits. Elevated Legs-Up-the-Wall Pose reduces the systemic effects of stress. It quiets the mind and refreshes the heart and lungs. It is especially beneficial for those who have varicose veins, who stand for long periods, who tend to retain water, or whose legs swell easily.

Cautions

- This pose is not recommended for those who should avoid inversions: individuals with hiatal hernias, eye pressure, retinal problems, heart problems, neck problems, and menstruating women. If you have any concerns about practicing inverted poses, consult your health care professional.
- Some people find this pose difficult for their lower back, particularly in the beginning. If this occurs, bend your knees and place your feet on the wall or cross your ankles loosely and let the wall support your legs and feet.
- This pose is recommended for those with mild hypertension currently being controlled with medication. In fact, it can help to lower blood pressure.

Do not practice this pose:

- if it creates pressure in the head.
- if you are menstruating.
- after the third month of pregnancy or if at risk for miscarriage.
- if you have spondylolisthesis or spondylolysis.
- if you have a sinus infection. Inverted poses can make this condition worse, including forcing the infection into the eustachian tubes of the ear. However, if you have general stuffiness, this pose may help to clear your head.

Reclining Twist with a Bolster

Prop

- bolster

Optional Props

- single-fold blanket
- extra blanket for warmth
- clock or timer

At first glance, a twisting pose looks like we are tying ourselves up in knots. Doesn't life do that to us enough? you say. In fact, Reclining Twist with a Bolster is really a chance to untie the physical, emotional, and mental knots that we have been twisted into by living in this fast-paced world.

In this pose, you sit on the floor with a bolster at your side; as you twist toward the bolster, you lean on it until it supports your weight. Reclining Twist with a Bolster stretches the muscles of the entire back and makes a pleasant transition from the back-bending of the previous poses to the forward bending of the poses that follow.

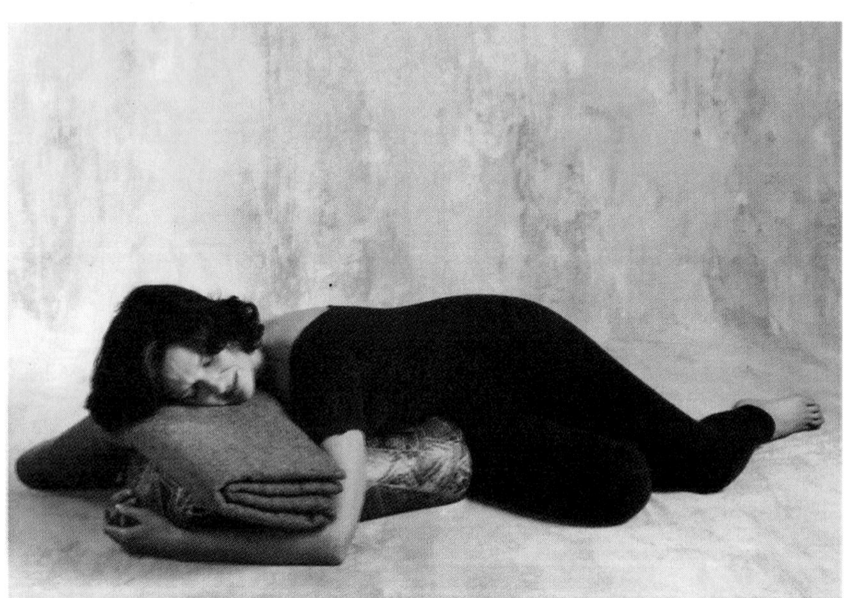

FIGURE 5.6
Reclining Twist with a Bolster

Setting Up. Sit on the floor with your right hip close to the end of the bolster. Bend your knees and slide your feet to the left, so the outside of your right leg rests on the floor. Your left leg can rest on your right leg, or you can open the space between them, whichever is more comfortable. Turn to your right, and put your hands on the floor, one on either side of the bolster. Gently press your hands into the floor to lengthen the front of your body. Then bend your elbows and lower yourself onto the bolster. Place your arms on the floor in a comfortable position.

In this position, your upper back turns toward the right, and your knees point in the opposite direction, giving a light twist to the vertebral column. To increase the twist, turn your head to the right, away from your knees. If this feels like too much, either rest your forehead on the bolster or turn your head toward your knees. You may want to place a single-fold blanket under your head for support.

Being There. Rest on the bolster. Relax the space between your shoulder blades. Use each exhalation as a reminder to release into the twist and onto the bolster. Let yourself feel longer and longer over the bolster, and increase the twist based upon this feeling of elongation. Breathe quietly.

Coming Back. Practice Reclining Twist with a Bolster for an equal amount of time on each side: one to two minutes, depending on your comfort and your level of experience. Come out of the pose carefully to avoid any strain on your back. First, turn your head toward your knees and rest for 1 or 2 breaths. Place your palms on the floor under your shoulders. Press down with your hands as you slowly sit up. Move your props to the other side and repeat the pose.

Benefits. Reclining Twist with a Bolster relieves stress in the back muscles and those along the sides of the body. It also helps to stretch the intercostals (the muscles between the ribs). As all the muscles relax, breathing is enhanced.

Caution

- This pose can be done by most people, even those with severe back problems. If you have spondylolisthesis, spondylolysis, disc disease, or chronic sacroiliac problems, proceed very carefully.

My heart gives thanks—
for empty moments
given to dreams.
—William S. Braithwaite

Supported Seated-Angle Pose

Prop

- bolster

Optional Props

- chair
- 1 or more single-fold blankets
- towel
- extra blanket for warmth
- clock or timer

This sitting pose is traditionally used to stretch the legs. I recommend that even very flexible individuals practice this supported variation to enhance relaxation. You do not have to work aggressively to achieve the physiological benefits of the pose.

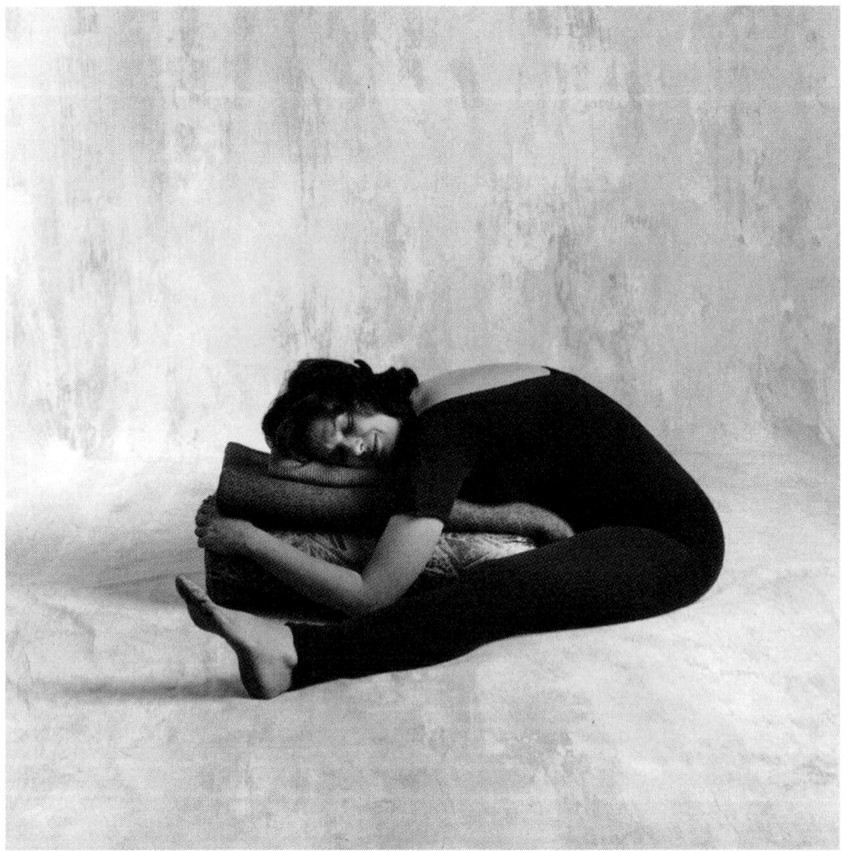

FIGURE 5.7 Supported Seated-Angle Pose

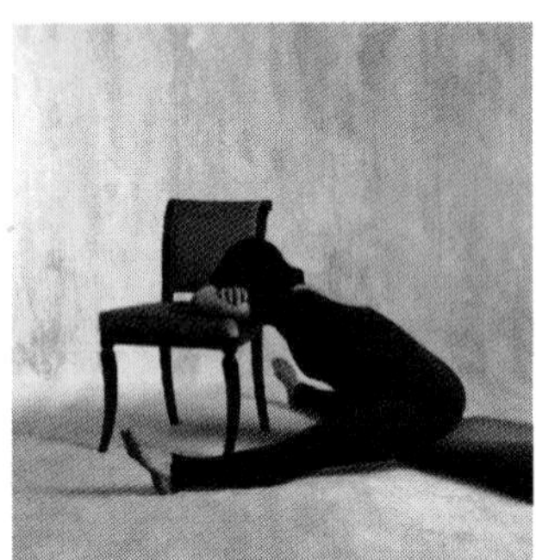

FIGURE 5.8 Supported Seated-Angle Pose, Variation

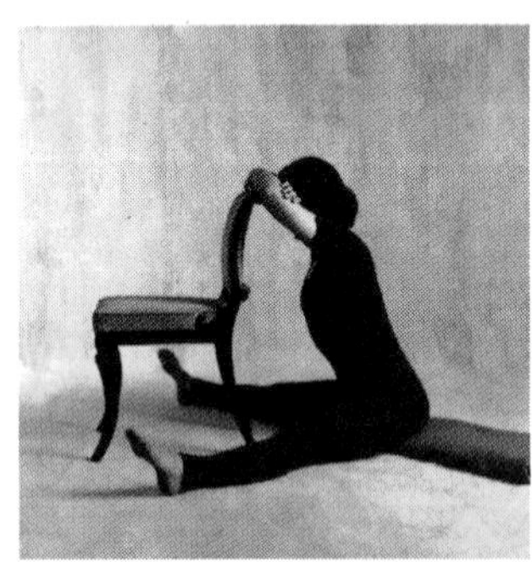

FIGURE 5.9 Supported Seated-Angle Pose, Variation

Setting Up. Sit on the floor, with your legs apart and the bolster between them. Do not position your legs so far apart that you overstretch your inner knees. If you feel inner knee discomfort, bring your legs closer together until the discomfort subsides and you feel the stretch only in your inner thighs. Whether you feel discomfort in one inner knee or both, bring both legs in, so each is the same distance from the midline of the body.

If you can maintain the natural inward curve of your lumbar spine, located at the level of your waist, you can proceed. If your lower back rounds, sit on the corner of a single-fold blanket. This will lift the pelvis and tip it forward to maintain the lumbar curve. Feel free to increase the height of your blanket so you can lean forward without strain.

Once comfortably seated, lean forward and rest your torso, arms, and head on the bolster. There are three possible positions for your arms and head. As always, experiment and select what feels best to you. You can:

- fold your arms and rest your forehead on them or turn your head to one side;
- let your arms rest on the bolster, folded or separated, free from your head; or
- rest your head on the bolster and let your arms rest on the floor, alongside the bolster.

Relax your neck and throat. Move your chin slightly toward your chest, so the back of your neck is long.

Remember, the point of this pose is not to stretch, but to open. If you are less flexible and cannot rest easily on the bolster, come up and increase the height of the support by adding 1 or more single-fold blankets. You can also place a folded towel under your head. Another option: Use a chair. You can lean forward and rest on the seat. Add 1 or more single-fold blankets to the chair seat until you are comfortable. If this is still too stressful, turn the chair around and rest against its back.

As with all forward bends, Supported Seated-Angle Pose can strain your lower back. Usually this is alleviated by sitting on a support high enough to tip the pelvis forward. For some people, however, the sacroiliac joint is still aggravated. Sacroiliac aggravation is experienced most often as a circle of pain about the size of a quarter or fifty-cent piece over the left or the right side of the sacrum.

If you feel sacroiliac pain in this pose, you may find relief by adjusting your body slightly asymmetrically to the bolster or chair. Twist your body slightly to one side and lean forward again. If this does not relieve the pain or aggravates it, twist slightly to the other side. If neither adjustment relieves the pain or discomfort, skip this pose and seek the advice of your health care professional regarding your sacroiliac alignment. If you are able to proceed, close your eyes.

Movement never lies.
—Martha Graham

Being There. Breathe normally. Let your body be completely supported by the props. Feel the sensations of your body, as the external world fades away. Imagine you are entering a temple, where you can lay down your burdens and rest in the stillness. There are no demands on you now. Let your abdomen and chest soften, as you breathe easily and freely.

Coming Back. Practice Supported Seated-Angle Pose for 3 to 5 minutes; those with more experience can stay up to 10 minutes. When you feel ready, open your eyes and rest for a few breaths. Place your hands on the bolster or chair, and use the strength of your arms to slowly sit up. Place your hands behind you, and lean back to relieve your back.

We have so many words for states of mind, and so few for the states of the body.
—JEANNE MOREAU

Benefits. In general, forward-bending poses quiet the organs of digestion and elimination, such as the stomach, intestines, and liver. Women often find this pose especially pleasant during their menstrual cycle and throughout pregnancy. If you are pregnant, make sure there is room between the chair and your belly, so you and the baby are comfortable. In addition, this pose balances the squeezing effect on the spine and kidneys that back-bending poses create. As a counterbalancing movement to back bends, this pose opens the lower back area. Supported Seated-Angle Pose calms mental agitation and can be practiced to relieve headaches (see chapter 8) or insomnia (see chapter 9).

Cautions

- Take the utmost care to create comfort for your neck, lower back, and knees in Supported Seated-Angle Pose. If you experience discomfort in any of these areas after experimenting with prop height and placement, do not practice this pose.
- If you experience any neck pain or discomfort during or after the pose, make sure that the neck does not sag but that you maintain the normal cervical curve, as you would when standing upright.
- If you experience pain or discomfort in one or both inner knees, bring your legs closer together, as described in Setting Up. If pain persists, do not pactice the pose for a few days and then try it again. If you still experience the pain or discomfort, consult your health care professional.
- If you have disc disease in your lower back or chronic sacroiliac dysfunction, lower the height of the props under your sitting bones and raise the height under your head and chest.
- You should not feel any sacroiliac pain or discomfort. If you do, try the adjustments described in Setting Up. If they fail to alleviate the discomfort, skip this pose for now.

Supported Crossed-Legs Pose

This is another relaxing seated pose, similar to the previous one, except that the legs are crossed at the ankles in a relaxed tailor position. In yoga we are taught that the nervous system benefits from keeping the poses as symmetrical as possible. In Supported Crossed-Legs Pose, we practice first with the right ankle on top of the left ankle and then reverse the cross for an equal amount of time. In so doing, the hemispheres of the brain receive an equal amount of input from the nerves that interpret our spatial position. The brain translates this feedback as quietness.

Prop

- chair

Optional Props

- 1 or more single-fold blankets
- nonskid mat
- extra blanket for warmth
- clock or timer

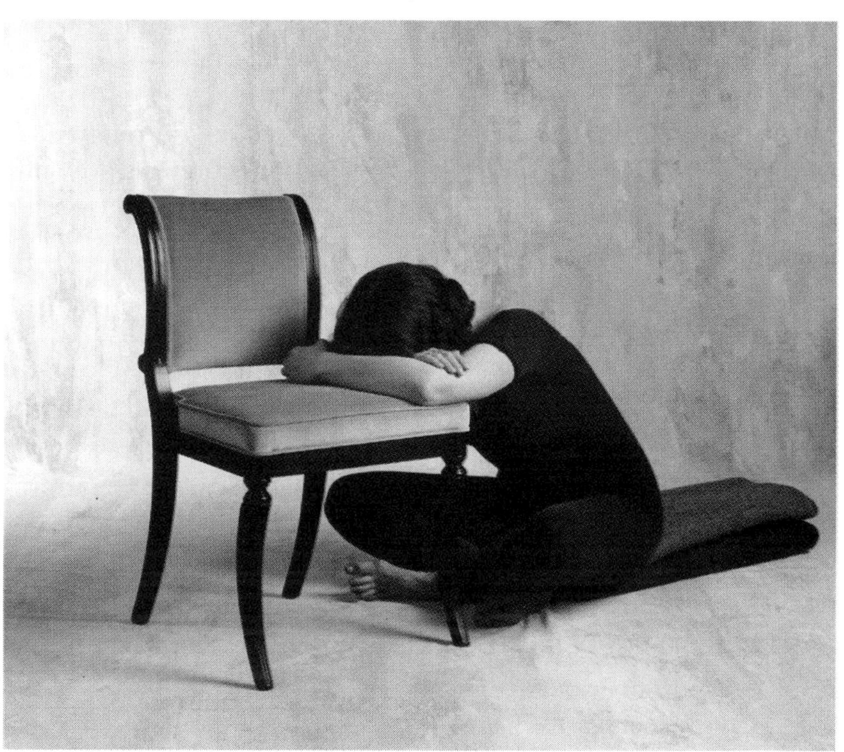

FIGURE 5.10 Supported Crossed-Legs Pose

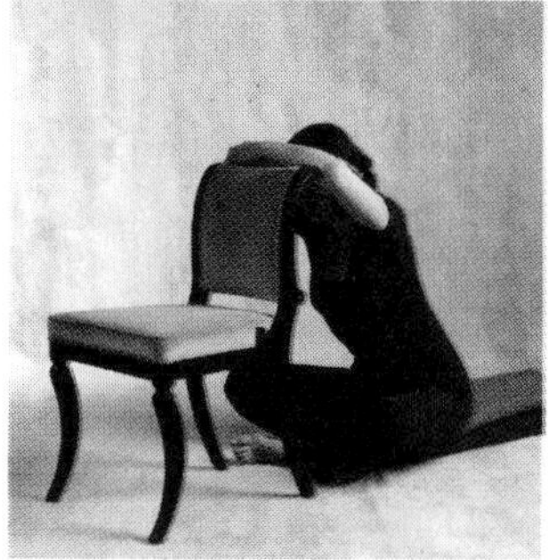

FIGURE 5.11 Supported Crossed-Legs Pose, Variation

Setting Up. Sit on the floor with the chair in front of you. Take care that the chair does not slide. If it does, place it on a nonskid mat. Cross your legs at your ankles. If you can maintain the natural inward curve of your lumbar spine, located at the level of your waist, you can proceed. If your lower back rounds, sit on the corner of one or more single-fold blankets. This will lift the pelvis and tip it forward to create the inward lumbar curve.

If you know that you can bend forward easily, you can practice this pose with the chair seat facing you. If you do not bend forward easily, place 1 or more single-fold blankets to raise the height of the seat, or turn the chair so its back faces you. These variations will allow you to come forward as you maintain the natural curves of the spine.

Come forward, fold your arms, and rest them on the chair. Adjust the chair so that you actually lean on it. If you bend forward easily, you might prefer having the chair farther from you. Whatever the distance, make sure that your lower back is lengthened.

Now rest your forehead on your arms, or turn your head to one side. Your neck should not sag when you rest the forehead on your folded arms. If it does, it means that your chin is moving up and out. To correct this, draw your chin slightly back and in. You can also add more prop height under your forehead. Close your eyes.

Being There. Breathe and enjoy the stillness, from without and within. Let the weight of your head rest completely. Breathe into your back, as you let it softly round. Feel as if all your problems roll off you, from the top your head and down your back. Remain present in the here and now.

Coming Back. Practice Supported Crossed-Legs Pose for 3 to 5 minutes. Remember to come up, reverse the cross of your ankles, and repeat the pose for equal time with the opposite ankle on top. To conclude, come up slowly and lean back on your hands to relieve your lower back. If you feel any discomfort in your back, lie on the floor with your calves resting on the the chair seat for a few minutes.

If you want to draw a bird,
you must become a bird.
—Hokusai

Benefits. Supported Crossed-Legs Pose is similar to Supported Seated Angle Pose, offering additional benefit to the lower abdomen. In Seated Angle Pose, the breath is felt more in the upper lungs. The breath moves differently in Supported Crossed-Legs Pose, and awareness is brought to the lower abdomen. Since most of us hold tension in the belly, this pose helps to release below the level of the navel. In addition, this pose cools and relaxes the digestive and reproductive organs, kidneys, and liver.

Cautions

- At no time should you feel any back discomfort or pain. If you do, come out of the pose and raise the height of your props. If this adjustment fails to relieve your discomfort, skip the pose for now.
- Do not practice this pose if you have diagnosed sacroiliac dysfunction, disc disease, spondylolisthesis, or spondylolysis.

Basic Relaxation Pose with Legs Elevated

The last pose in the Relax and Renew series is Basic Relaxation Pose with Legs Elevated, a variation of the basic pose to release tension in your lower back. Remember, while Basic Relaxation Pose is beneficial on its own, even deeper levels of relaxation are achieved if it is practiced at the conclusion of a longer restorative series.

Props
- standard-fold blanket
- 2 or more single-fold blankets
- eyebag

Optional Props
- sandbag
- extra blanket for warmth
- clock or timer

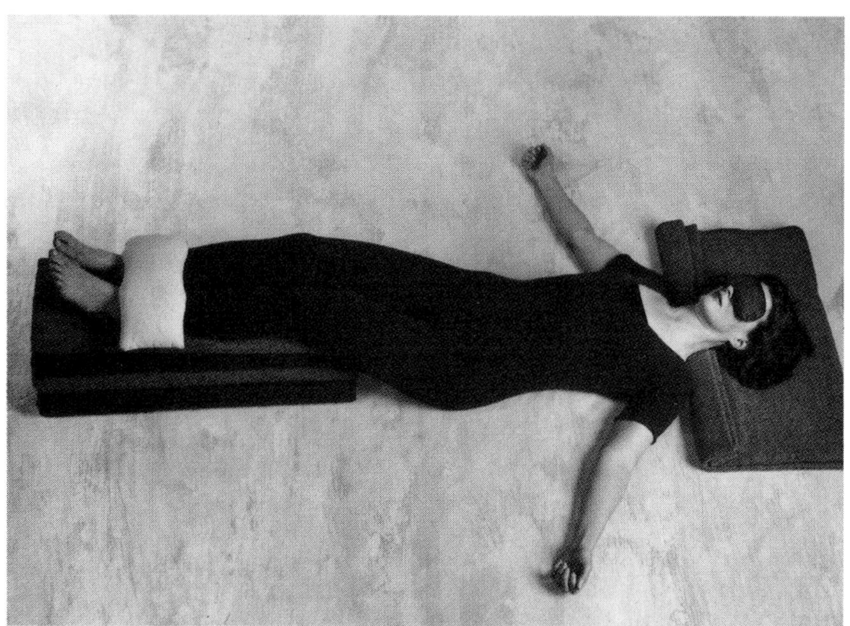

FIGURE 5.12 Basic Relaxation Pose with Legs Elevated

Setting Up. See page 25 for a complete description of Basic Relaxation Pose. As in the basic pose, before you lie down, position a standard-fold blanket for your head and neck to rest on. In this variation, you also stack two or more single-fold blankets to elevate your lower legs at least 10 to 12 inches and support their length.

Begin by sitting on the floor and placing your lower legs on the stack of single-fold blankets. You can place a sandbag across your ankles to anchor your legs on the blankets. If you have a tendency to get cold, cover your legs with an unfolded blanket. Use the strength and support of your arms to help you lie back.

Roll the long edge of your standard-fold blanket slightly to support the gentle curve of your neck. Adjust the prop placement under your head and neck so you are comfortable. Your chin should be slightly lower than your forehead. This position quiets the frontal lobes of the brain. If you are using an extra blanket for warmth, pull it up to cover your torso and arms. Cover your eyes with an eyebag. Rest your arms by the sides of your body.

Being There. See page 26 for a full discussion of being in Basic Relaxation Pose. In this variation, pay particular attention to your lower back. Let it sink downward, and allow any tension to be absorbed by the floor. Feel a release in the muscles of the lower back, and send this part of your body permission to let go.

Let your attention rest on the easy rise and fall of the abdomen with each breath. When you feel ready, begin the Centering Breath (see pages 24 and 26) and repeat for up to 10 breaths. Be sure to leave some time for normal breathing before coming out of the pose.

Coming Back. Practice Basic Relaxation Pose for 5 to 20 minutes. To come out of the pose, slide your legs out from under the sandbag if you are using one. Slowly bend one knee, then the other, and roll onto your side. Let the eyebag fall off by itself. Gradually open your eyes. Rest in this position for a few breaths. To sit up, press the floor with the elbow of your lower arm and the palm of the hand of your upper arm. Take a few breaths before standing up and resuming your normal activities.

Benefits. The lower back is especially vulnerable if you sit a lot or have weak abdominal muscles. Practicing this variation of Basic Relaxation Pose helps to relieve tension in your abdomen, as well as any tension in your lower back from the back-bending restorative poses. The elevation of the legs reduces fatigue from standing or sitting for long periods of time.

Caution

- If you are more than three months pregnant, practice Side-Lying Relaxation Pose (see chapter 13).

Wisdom is the ability to see life as it is, not the way I want it to be.
—Charlotte Joko Beck

PRACTICE SUMMARY

Here is a summary of the Relax and Renew series for easy reference. It will take between 60 and 90 minutes to do the whole series. If your time is limited, see chapter 6, where you will find shorter programs for home, work, or on the go.

60 to 90 Minutes

POSE	TIME
Simple Supported Back Bend	1 to 5 minutes
Supported Bound-Angle Pose	10 to 15 minutes
Mountain Brook Pose	5 to 7 minutes
Supported Bridge Pose	15 minutes
Elevated Legs-Up-the-Wall Pose	15 minutes
Reclining Twist with a Bolster	3 minutes
Supported Seated-Angle Pose	3 to 5 minutes
Supported Crossed-Legs Pose	3 to 5 minutes
Basic Relaxation Pose with Legs Elevated	5 to 20 minutes

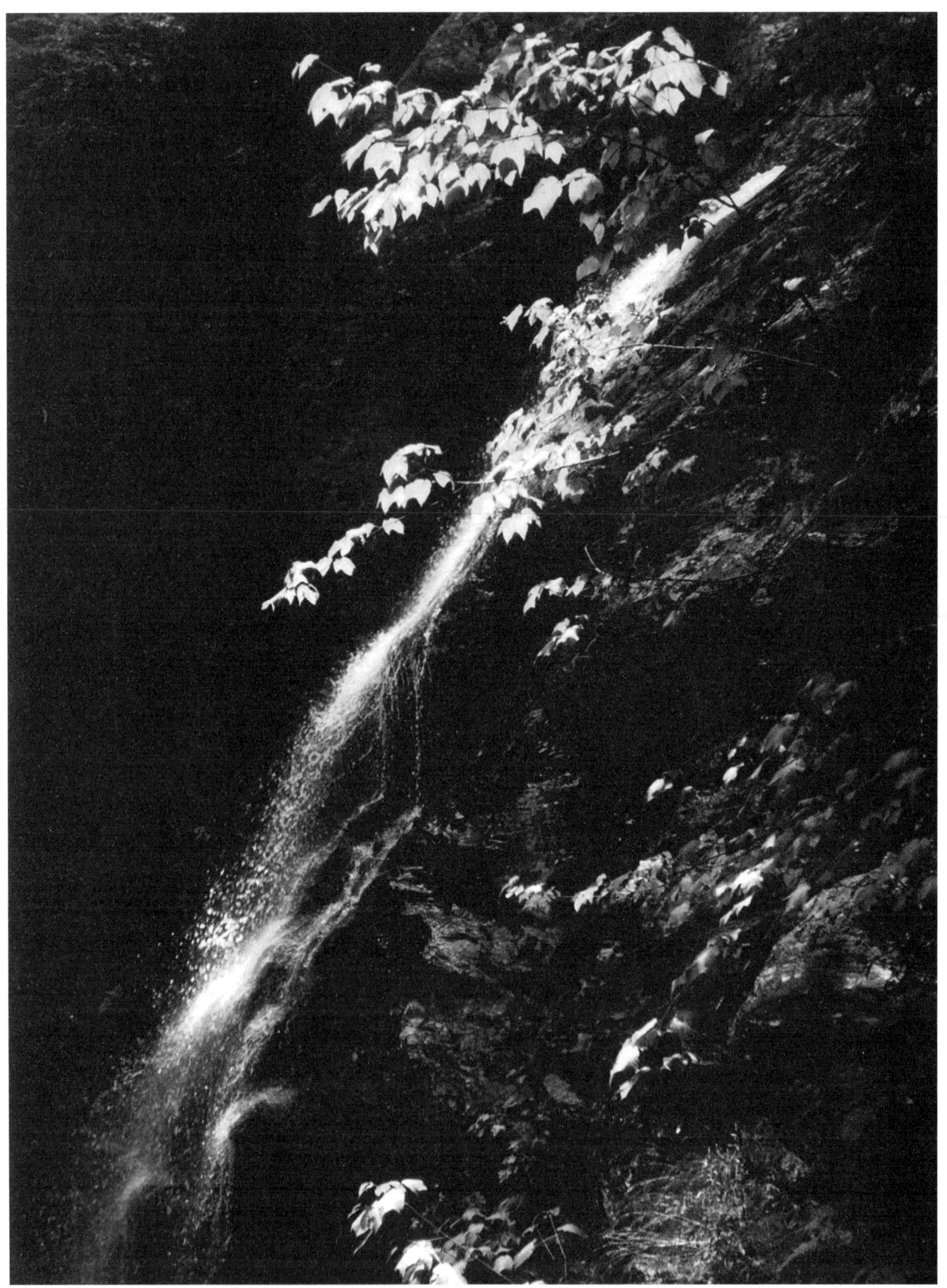

CHAPTER SIX

BUSY DAYS

Poses for Times When There's No Time

IN A PERFECT WORLD, we would all have time for a long restorative yoga practice daily. But obligations to work, family, friends, and community often leave us with little time for self-care. It is precisely when we are the most stressed that we need to relax and renew ourselves. This chapter describes three series that bring restorative yoga into your busy life. The first one you can practice at home or on vacation; the second is for the office; the third is for when you're on the go.

The 15-Minute Relaxation. To relax deeply in this amount of time, you must have a quiet room, but you can get by with a minimum of props. There are only three poses: Legs-Up-the-Wall Pose, Supported Child's Pose, and Basic Relaxation Pose. Practice them in the order presented. As always, I have listed a full complement of optional props. If you can't find even 15 minutes, practice Basic Relaxation Pose for 5.

Better Than a Coffee Break. Some of the most stressful times are at work. These two restorative poses need a chair and desk (or table) and together take only 5 minutes.

The Totally Invisible Relaxation. This relaxation technique will serve you well. I have practiced it in taxis and airplanes, at the theater, and even at parties. Use it when you need it, right where you are.

Legs-Up-the-Wall Pose

Prop

- wall

Optional Props

- standard-fold blanket
- eyebag
- clock or timer

This pose is simple to practice, even when traveling. Just lie on your back, and let a nearby wall support your legs. This pose brings the blood and lymph fluid to pool in the abdomen, refreshing the leg muscles and enhancing the health of the circulatory system. In addition, the pose reverses the energy of the legs from moving down and out to the feet, as in our normal stance, to moving down and back to the pelvis. Nothing feels better to tired legs and feet than being elevated.

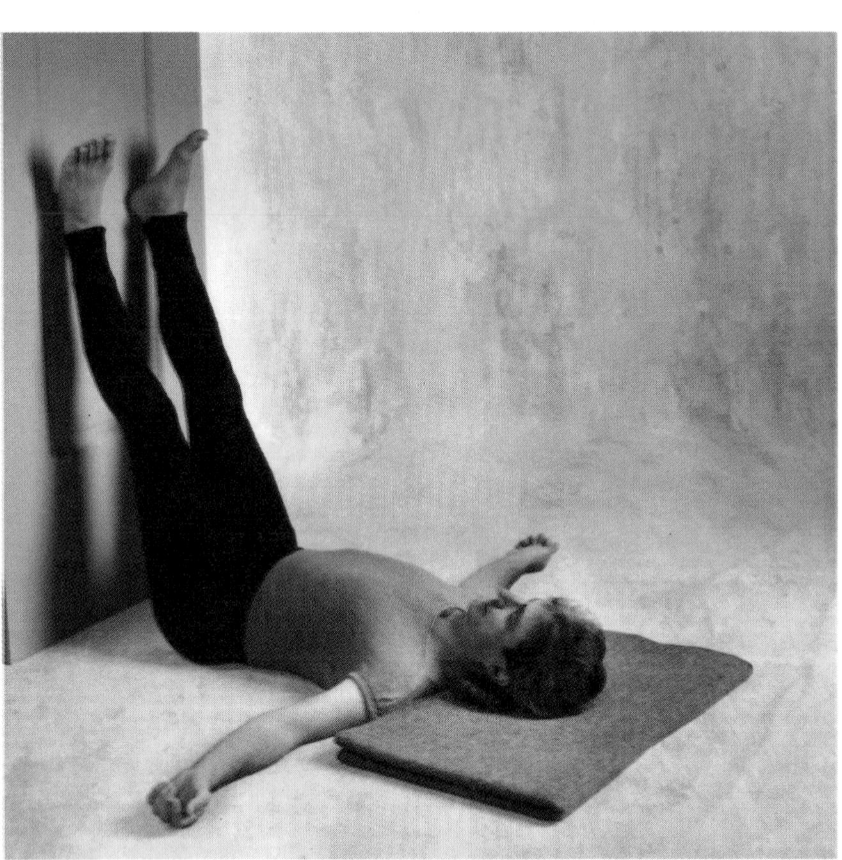

FIGURE 6.1
Legs-Up-the-Wall Pose

Setting Up. To begin, sit on the floor, with one shoulder near the wall and your thighs parallel to the wall. Roll back as you swing your legs up the wall. Once in position, make sure that your lower back is not rounded and your tailbone and buttocks are not lifting off the floor. If they are, move slightly away from the wall so that your lower back is comfortably supported by the floor.

If your chin lifts toward the ceiling, place a standard-fold blanket under your head and neck to support your cervical curve. Make sure your chin is slightly lower than your forehead, but do not force your chin down and flatten the back of your neck.

Keep your legs straight, but relaxed. Place your arms out to your sides, with the palms turned up. Close your eyes. Place an eyebag over them.

Being There. Take several long, slow breaths. As you do, imagine the fluid in your legs flowing down toward the abdomen. With it, all tension drains out of your legs. They begin to feel lighter and softer. Imagine that your brain is shrinking in size, as it moves away from your forehead and sinks toward the back of your head and the floor. Feel your entire spine supported by the floor. The position of the arms creates a feeling of being open and free. Enjoy this feeling.

Coming Back. Practice Legs-Up-the-Wall Pose for 5 minutes. When ready, remove the eyebag and open your eyes. Rest for a few breaths before bending your knees toward your chest and rolling to one side. Pause again for a few breaths before slowly coming to a sitting position with the help of your arms.

Benefits. Legs-Up-the-Wall Pose reduces swelling and fatigue in the legs.

Cautions

- If you experience strain at the back of your knees in this pose, try these variations. Move closer to the wall so that your legs are more perpendicular. If you are already close to the wall and the strain persists, bend your knees several inches. If these adjustments do not alleviate the strain, move about 12 inches away from the wall and bend your knees, resting the soles of your feet on the wall.
- If you have lower back pain in this pose, move about 12 inches away from the wall and bend your knees, resting the soles of your feet on the wall.
- This pose is recommended for those with mild hypertension currently being controlled with medication. In fact, it can help to lower blood pressure.
- If you have any concerns about practicing inverted poses, consult your health care professional.

Do not practice this inverted pose:

- if you have a hiatal hernia.
- if you are menstruating.
- if you are more than three months pregnant or at risk for miscarriage.
- if you have sciatica.

Make haste slowly.
—Caesar Augustus

Supported Child's Pose

Prop

- bolster

Optional Props

- 1 or more single-fold blankets
- 2 towels
- sandbag
- long-roll blanket
- extra blanket for warmth
- clock or timer

Supported Child's Pose is the familiar posture of rest and sleep for babies and young children. When you practice this pose, not only will it help to relieve tension in your lower back, but it may evoke a sense of security from your earliest days. This pose is one of introversion, of curling up and reconnecting with feelings of support and release.

Setting Up. Begin by kneeling on a carpeted floor or blanket, with your knees hip-width apart and your bolster in front of you. Use more padding under your knees and shins if you need it. To avoid stress on the ligaments of your outer ankles, point your toes directly backward and not toward each other. Sit back on your heels.

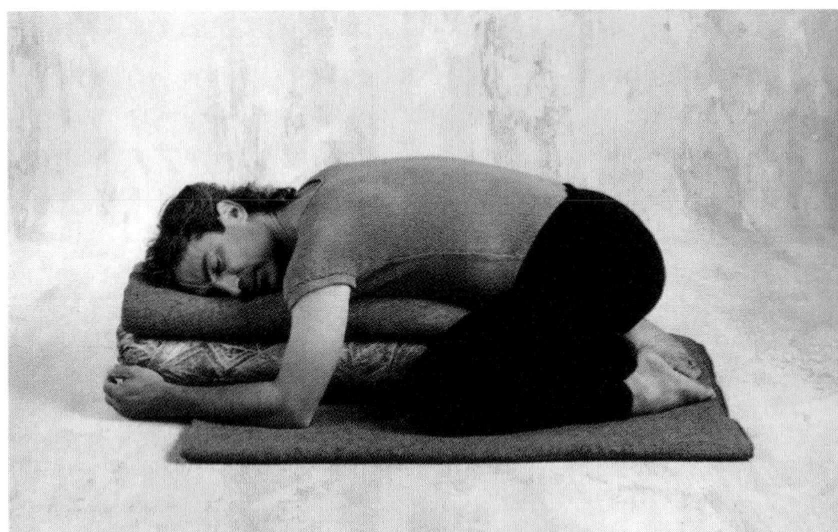

FIGURE 6.2
Supported Child's Pose

If you experience discomfort in your knees, ankles, or tops of your feet, come up and try one or both of the following adjustments. Place one towel, folded lengthwise, into the bend of your knees to create more space in the knee joints. Place the other towel, rolled lengthwise, under the front of the ankles, and let your feet hang over the roll. Experiment with the thickness of these folded and rolled towels to get them just right for you.

Sit back on your heels again. Separate your knees wide enough to place the bolster between your thighs. To enhance relaxation, hold a sandbag across your lower back as you bend forward. The weight of the bag helps to relax the muscles of your lower back.

Your torso should be completely supported by the bolster and your thighs. Your chest should rest easily on the bolster. Let your tailbone drop toward your heels. This action will lengthen your lower back as you relax. Your buttocks do not have to touch your heels.

If you need more support, try one of the following variations. Come up to a kneeling position and place a long-roll blanket on your heels and sit back, or come to a kneeling position and significantly raise the height of your torso support by adding 1 or more single-fold blankets. If you have difficulty breathing, push the bolster forward so it only supports your breastbone and lets your belly hang free.

Turn your head to one side, and bring your chin slightly toward your chest. Turn your head to the opposite side halfway through the practice of the pose. If the side head position is uncomfortable, rest on your forehead and slightly tuck your chin toward your chest. Make sure you can breathe easily regardless of your head position.

Place your arms so that they either reach back toward your feet or forward around the edges of the bolster. The position of the arms is unimportant; it is important that you are comfortable. Close your eyes.

Being There. Take several slow breaths. As you do, let your shoulders move away from the ears. Let your belly relax and feel supported. The counter-pressure of the bolster on the belly may feel especially good if you have menstrual cramps.

Coming Back. Practice Supported Child's Pose for 3 minutes. Be sure that you spend equal time with your head turned in both directions. Open your eyes. Reach back with one hand and slide the sandbag off your back and to one side. Place your palms on the floor, under your shoulders. Press your hands into the floor, inhale, and sit up slowly onto your heels. Rest for a moment. Come to a kneeling position and immediately bring one leg forward, placing your foot on the floor. Press your hands on the forward thigh, and inhale deeply as you come to a standing position. Coming out of the pose in this way prevents discomfort in the knees.

Be careful when in a hurry.
—JAMAICAN PROVERB

Benefits. Supported Child's Pose gently stretches the lower back, relieves shoulder tension, and quiets the mind.

Cautions

- To protect the knees, ankles, and feet, follow the suggestions in the Setting Up and Coming Back sections.

Do not practice this pose:

- if you have a chronic back condition, including but not limited to spondylolisthesis, spondylolysis, spinal stenosis, disc disease, nerve symptoms (such as radiating pain or numbness, or difficulties with bowel or bladder function).

- if you are more than three months pregnant.

Basic Relaxation Pose

Prop

- standard-fold blanket

Optional Props

- eyebag
- long-roll blanket or bolster
- blanket or pillow to prop heels
- extra blanket for warmth
- clock or timer

As explained in chapter 4, this pose is the heart of restorative practice. Relaxing completely, even if it is only for 5 minutes, is one of the most important skills you can acquire. When you have learned to relax whenever and wherever you need to, you can use this skill in a variety of situations to reduce stress and its accompanying fatigue.

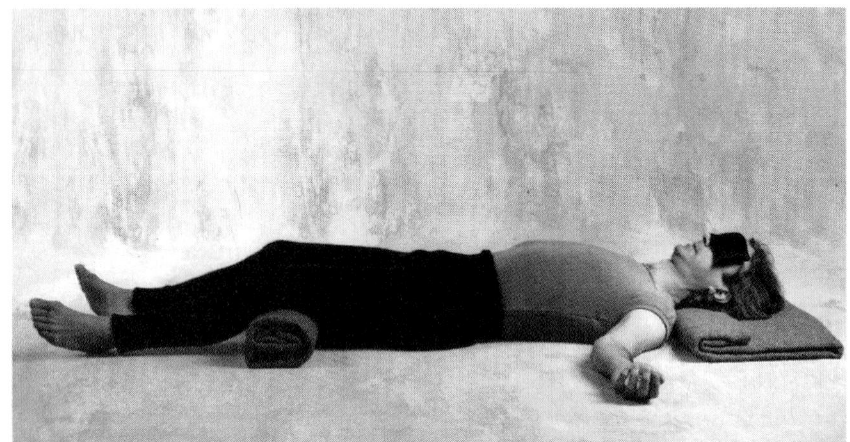

FIGURE 6.3
Basic Relaxation Pose

Setting Up, Being There, and Coming Back. Refer to page 25 for full instructions. Practice Basic Relaxation Pose for 7 minutes.

Benefits. All the physiological measures of stress are reduced by a period of deep relaxation. Fatigue is diminished and life is just easier to handle when you are more relaxed.

Caution

- If you are more than three months pregnant, practice Side-Lying Relaxation Pose (see chapter 13).

Desk Forward Bend

I remember how restful it was during my school days to lean forward and rest my head and folded arms on my desk. Try this pose at your desk or in the lunchroom at work or school.

Props

- desk or table
- chair

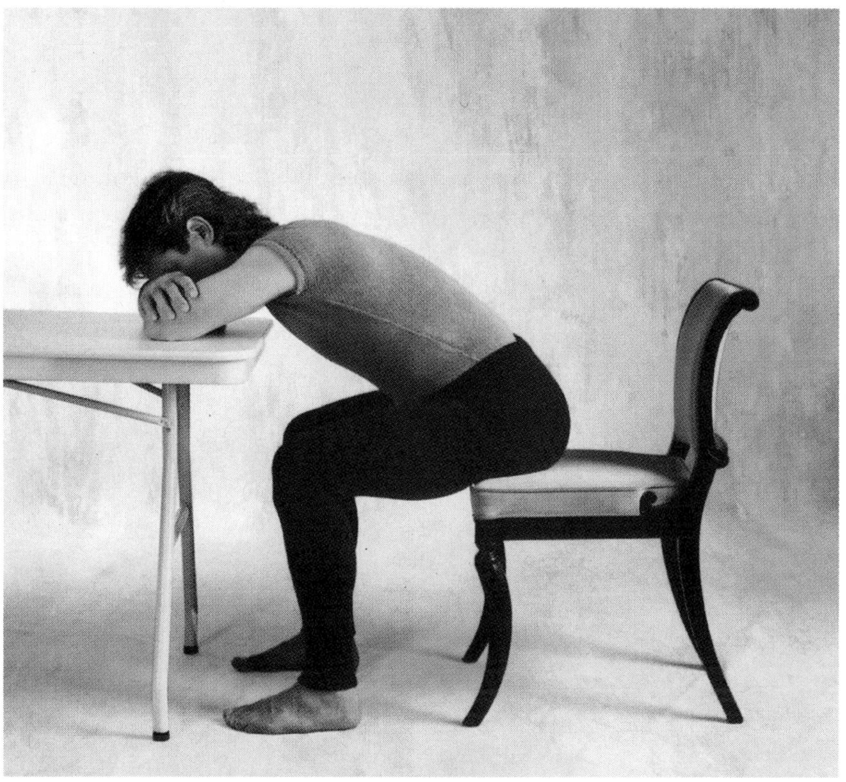

FIGURE 6.4
Desk Forward Bend

Setting Up. Place your chair (without rollers) near your desk so that you can easily lean forward. Sit at the edge of the chair seat, with your feet flat on the floor. Lean forward and place your folded arms on the desk, so you feel securely supported. Rest your forehead on your arms. Tilt your chin slightly toward your chest. Close your eyes.

Being There. Breathe slowly and deeply for the first few breaths, then resume normal breathing. Let the desk support your arms, your head, and your cares. Let the next few minutes of relaxation fill you.

Coming Back. Practice Desk Forward Bend for 3 minutes. To come up, unfold your arms as you lift your head. Inhale, and press your hands into the desk to help you return to sitting. Sit in your chair for one more long, slow breath before moving on to the next pose or on with your day.

Caution

- Take care of your neck and lower back in this pose. When you are forward, make sure your chin is tucked close to your body. Come up slowly to protect your lower back.

Chair Forward Bend

Prop

- chair

This pose is another supported forward bend, but this time you rest on your thighs instead of the desk. Chair Forward Bend provides the double benefit of a forward bend and a mild inversion.

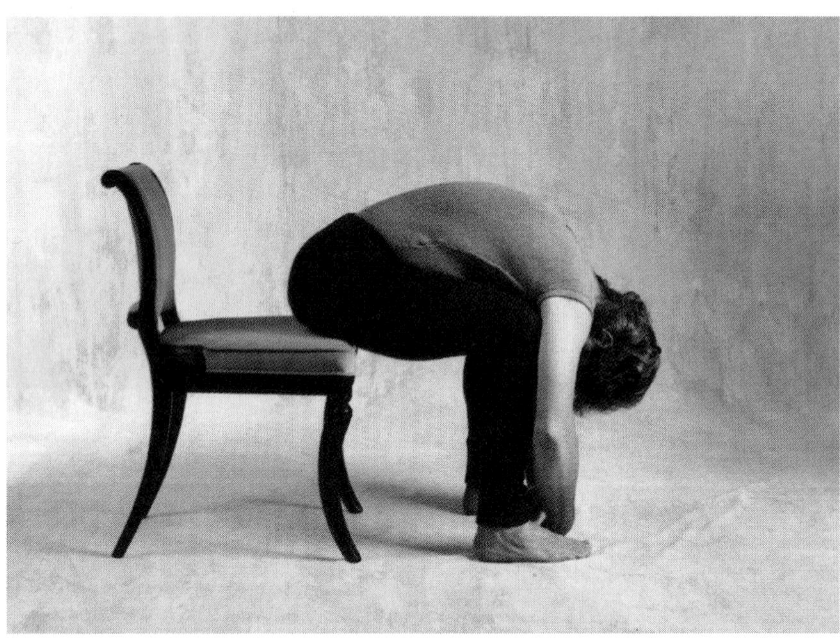

FIGURE 6.5
Chair Forward Bend

Setting Up. Select a stable chair that does not roll, and position it away from your desk. Sit near the edge of the chair seat, with your feet firmly on the floor and about 6 to 10 inches apart. Slowly bend forward until your chest rests on your thighs. Let your head hang down naturally. Allow your arms to dangle by your sides. Close your eyes.

Being There. Breathe quietly. Let gravity stretch your back. Feel all tension in your shoulders melt away. Rest.

Coming Back. Practice Chair Forward Bend for 2 minutes. To come up, put your hands on the sides of the chair seat, and press down as you inhale and lift your torso. Once upright, take 2 slow breaths before returning to your day's activities.

Benefits. Chair Forward Bend stretches the lower back, relieves tension in the shoulders, and quiets the mind.

Cautions

Do not practice this pose:

- if you are more than three months pregnant.
- if you have a hiatal hernia, retinal problems, eye pressure, or a sinus infection.
- Proceed very carefully if you have diagnosed disc disease. If you have any questions about the appropriateness of this pose for you, consult your health care professional.

PRACTICE *The Totally Invisible Relaxation*

Optional Prop

- chair

There may be times when you need to practice restorative yoga poses but your situation does not permit it. Perhaps you are involved in a long business meeting or immersed in family responsibilities. With the Totally Invisible Relaxation, you can actually relax, just where you are, sitting or standing. The first step is to realize that you need to relax. If you have been practicing the restorative poses, you may find it easy to drop down into relaxation. If not, try it anyway. Your skills will improve with practice.

Setting Up. Bring your attention to the position of your body, especially your spine. Sit or stand with the spine long. Avoid rounding your lower back if you are sitting or slumping if you are standing. Ideally there should be a gentle concave arch at your back waist. (See chapter 16 for suggestions on good posture and chapter 17 for healthful sitting.)

Once you have positioned yourself with a long, gently curving spine, make sure that your head and neck are in line with the spine. Feel as if you are being gently lifted up by the crown of your head. Close your eyes, if your situation permits, or soften your gaze and look downward.

Being There. Gently bring your awareness to your breathing. Take several long and quiet breaths. If your breath seems stuck anywhere, it is likely that you have lost the lift of the spine. When the spine is lifted, your diaphragm can function at maximum efficiency and your breathing will feel easy.

As you exhale, let your shoulders drop away from your ears and your arms feel long and fluid. Let the hands and arms rest in your lap or on a table, or hang easily from the shoulders. Soften the abdomen and notice how it moves with your breathing. Release any tension around the eyes or in the jaw muscles. If sitting, your thighs are supported by the chair. If standing, keep your feet rooted to the floor, but don't overwork your legs.

Rest in the present moment. As you inhale and exhale, be who and where you are. Do not attempt to separate yourself from what is happening around you. Rather, be with what is, equally aware of your internal sensations as well as the external world. Notice the sounds in the room and the sounds outside the room. Feel the weight and texture of your clothes on your body. What is around you and in you is part of this perfect moment. Weave it into your relaxation.

Coming Back. When you have finished, take several more long, slow, silent breaths. Slowly open your eyes and allow your vision to come into focus. Return to the task at hand refreshed, optimistic, and present.

Benefits. The Totally Invisible Relaxation will enhance your ability to work, to create, and to interact with people and situations more skillfully.

Caution

- If you have low blood pressure, do not practice the standing variation for more than 2 minutes.

The body is shaped, disciplined, honored, and in time, trusted.
—MARTHA GRAHAM

PRACTICE SUMMARY

Here is a summary of the Busy Days practice options. As always, do what you can, and do it mindfully.

The 15-Minute Relaxation

POSE	TIME
Legs-Up-the-Wall Pose	5 minutes
Supported Child's Pose	3 minutes
Basic Relaxation Pose	7 minutes

Better Than a Coffee Break

POSE	TIME
Desk Forward Bend	3 minutes
Chair Forward Bend	2 minutes

The Totally Invisible Relaxation

POSE	TIME
Standing or Sitting	as needed

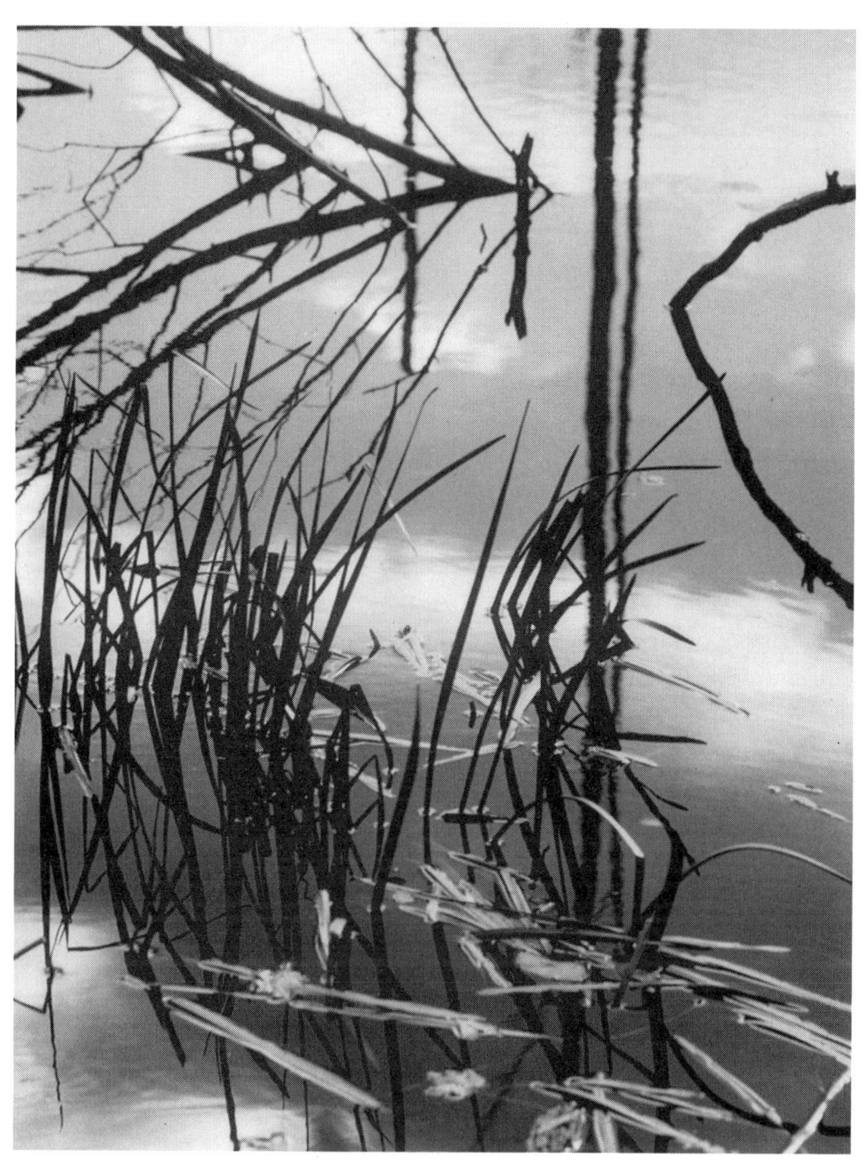

PART TWO: LIFE IN THE TWENTY-FIRST CENTURY

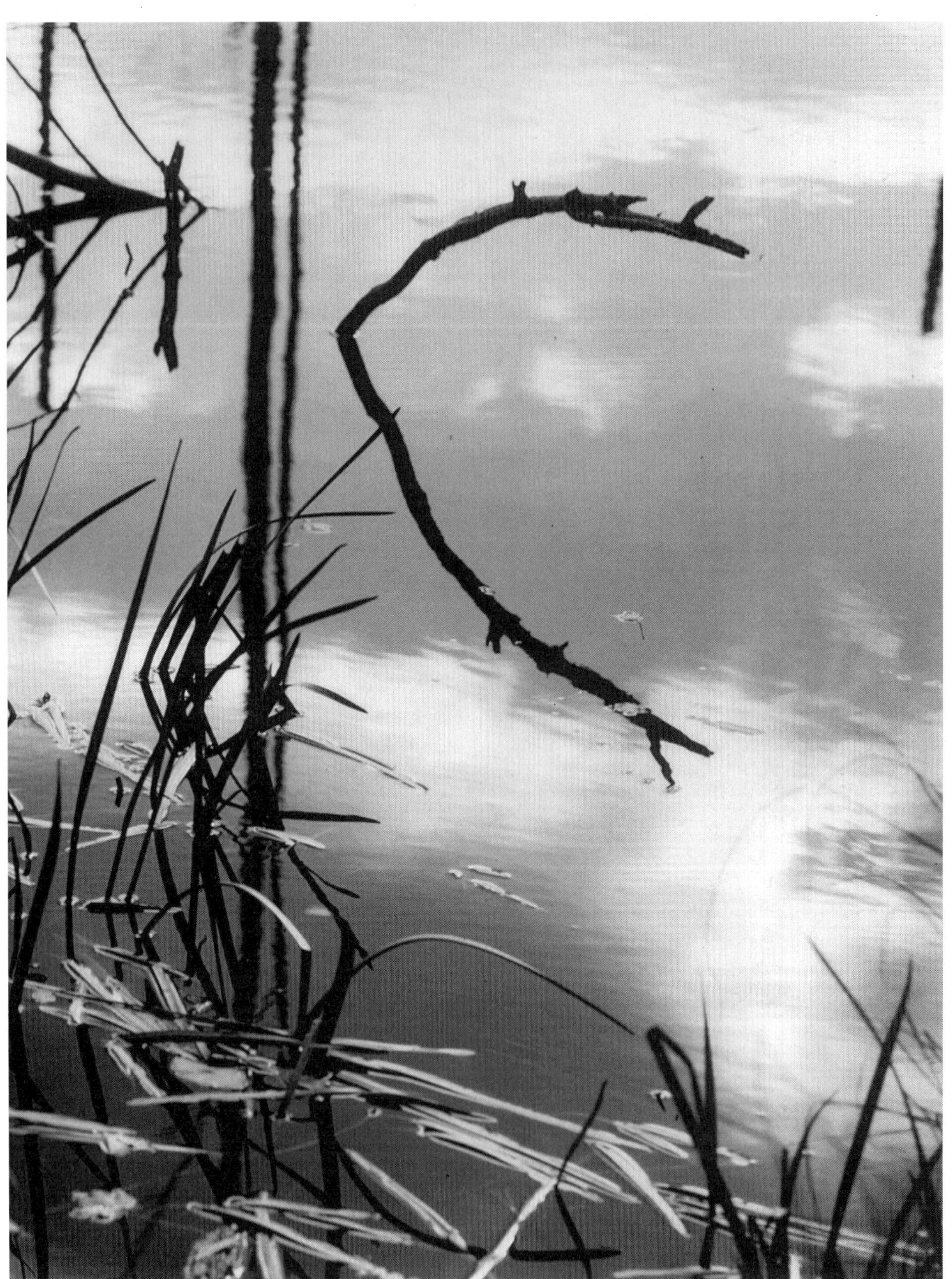

CHAPTER SEVEN

DOWN IN THE BACK

Poses for Lower Back Pain

LOWER BACK PAIN may be the price of being human and standing upright. A major health problem today, back pain ranks second only to the common cold as a reason for patients to visit a physician.[1] In many cases, back pain is due to overworked and misused muscles that go into spasm. These spasms can be so intense that they pull the spine out of alignment. Muscle spasm associated with lower back pain involves several factors, including posture, repetitive motion, weak abdominal muscles, and stress.

The most common contributor to lower back pain is bad posture. Most of us sit, stand, and move in ways that do not maintain the normal curves of the spinal column. Spinal muscles are forced to overwork to hold the body upright, creating muscular tension and ultimately lower back pain. (For a further discussion on how to stand and sit well, see chapters 16 and 17.)

Spinal muscles can also be stressed through repetitive motion. Consider the scientist bending over her microscope, the delivery person picking up packages, the tennis player practicing his serves. It is the habitual nature of these movements—constantly overusing some muscles and underusing others—that can lead to back pain.

Weak abdominal and lower back muscles contribute to spinal misalignments and poor body mechanics. The abdominal muscles wrap around the front and sides of the body in a basket-weave pattern. These muscles keep the discs in place during movement and

Glorify God in your body.
—I CORINTHIANS 20

support the natural curves of the spine, thus reducing stress on the spine during lifting, bending, and twisting.

Finally, stress plays its part in lower back pain. Under stress, our muscular tension is increased, and we pay less attention to healthy sitting, standing, walking, and lifting. This inattention can lead to injury.

The bad news: approximately 80 percent of adults will experience acute lower back pain during their lifetime. The good news: 90 percent will recover in a month on their own.[2] In the past, those with acute lower back pain turned to a variety of remedies, some more invasive than others. But current research indicates that the most useful approach to acute lower back pain is not extended bed rest, muscle relaxants, and surgery. Experts now recommend over-the-counter pain medications, such as acetaminophen and nonsteroidal anti-inflammatory drugs (NSAIDs); chiropractic treatment; and low-stress exercise, including swimming or walking.3 Among low-stress exercise techniques, I would include restorative yoga.

Down in the Back Series

The Down in the Back series can be practiced both for relief from lower back pain and to prevent pain from recurring. The series consists of six restorative yoga poses, beginning with two poses to relax the legs, abdomen, and lower back, and continuing with a supported back bend to stretch the front of the body and open the chest. These are followed by a supported twist to stretch and relieve tension in the small muscles of the lower back, and Supported Child's Pose to relax the abdomen and stretch the long muscles of the lower back. The series concludes with a variation of Basic Relaxation Pose, in which the lower legs rest on a chair seat and weight is placed on the abdomen. This practice takes 25 to 35 minutes.

Begin with a common-sense assessment of your symptoms. Be honest with yourself about how you feel, both physically and emotionally, and about what is possible for you. If you are in the middle of an attack, you probably will not feel like doing much. Try one of the shorter practice sessions at the end of this chapter. Familiarize yourself with chapters 3 and 4 and this chapter, especially the cautions, before you proceed.

Important Considerations

If you have lower back pain, consider the following before beginning this or any other exercise program.

Understand what is causing your back pain. The restorative yoga poses in this chapter are not a substitute for treatment by a health care professional. Do not begin this series, any other program in this book, or any exercise program until you have had an evaluation of your back condition by a health care professional.

Learn about the anatomy of your lower back. Located below the ribs and above the sacrum, the lower back consists of the bones of the spine itself, called the lumbar spine, and the surrounding muscles and ligaments. To help you understand the anatomy of this area, see chapter 16 for a thorough discussion of the spine.

Do what is possible to relieve the pain. If your back pain is associated with muscle and ligament strain and tension, you can practice the Down in the Back series. If you have chronic back conditions, including but not limited to spondylolisthesis, spondylolysis, spinal stenosis, disc disease, or nerve symptoms (such as, radiating pain or numbness, or difficulties with bowel or bladder function), consult a health care professional to discuss the appropriateness of restorative yoga for you.

Consult your health care professional if your back pain gets worse in intensity or duration after beginning the Down in the Back series or any other series in this book. Symptoms include: shooting pain down the back or side of one or both legs or in the groin area, numbness or weakness in your legs or arms, or loss of bowel or bladder control.

Total absence of humor renders life impossible.
—Colette

Practice yoga with care. Move slowly and mindfully, taking care not to aggravate your condition when coming into and out of the poses. Work with your position and your props until you feel comfortable. If a pose doesn't feel right, even after adjustments, move on to the next pose in the series or to a variation of Basic Relaxation Pose. If neither feels right, then find any position in which you are pain free—your sleeping position, for example—and use it to relax for up to 15 minutes. Try the series the next day.

Remember, with lower back pain some days will be easy, some more challenging. A pose may feel good one day and uncomfortable the next. Practice mindfully, and know that improvement is often a pattern of two steps forward and one step back. Consider your restorative practice a time to learn about your back and your limits, and take each setback as part of the learning process.

Strengthen your lower back and abdomen to prevent future problems. Once you are pain-free for six weeks, try the Relax and Renew series (in chapter 5). Read the Cautions section for each pose before you practice. Be willing to modify the pose even though you are pain-free.

As you find your way back to health, you may be ready to move on to more active yoga poses to strengthen and condition your abdomen and lower back. Try a private lesson or a yoga class with a teacher well-trained in helping students transition from modified poses for back pain to active poses. (See chapter 1 and Resources for tips on finding a teacher.) A regular walking program is another way to build strength. Use a common-sense approach to your walking, including good body mechanics, walking on level ground, appropriate shoes, and increasing your time and pace slowly.

Treat every body position, not just yoga poses, as an experiment. Pay particular attention to your body mechanics in sitting, standing, bending, lying, walking, carrying, lifting. See chapters 16 and 17 for helpful suggestions on sitting and standing.

Cautions

Do not practice this series:

- if you are menstruating and have back pain. Use the Moon Club series in chapter 12.
- if you are pregnant and have back pain. Use the Pea in the Pod series in Chapter 13.

There is no such thing as an accident. What we call by that name is the effect of some cause which we do not see.
—Voltaire

Hanging Dog Pose

In Downward-Facing Dog Pose, one of the most versatile yoga poses, you make an inverted V shape with your body, mimicking the stretch a dog takes when first rising from sleep. In the supported version, Hanging Dog Pose, you loop a belt around your hips and over a doorknob, and allow these props to support your body weight. As you hang, the abdomen relaxes. It is this feeling of letting go that brings relief when you have lower back pain.

Props

- nonskid mat
- belt
- door with doorknobs

Optional Props

- chair
- clock or timer

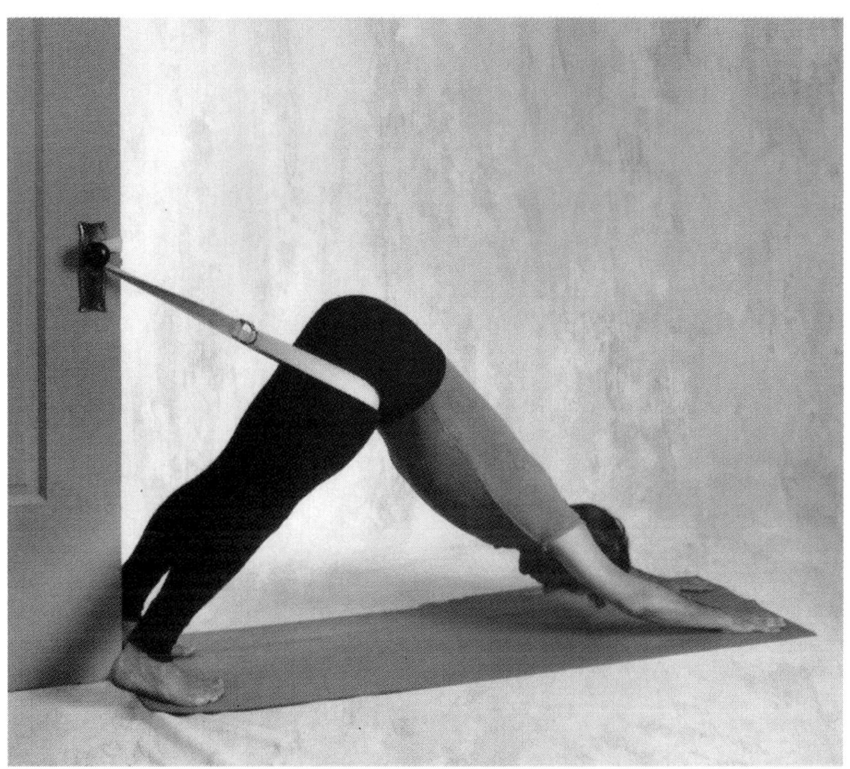

FIGURE 7.1 Hanging Dog Pose

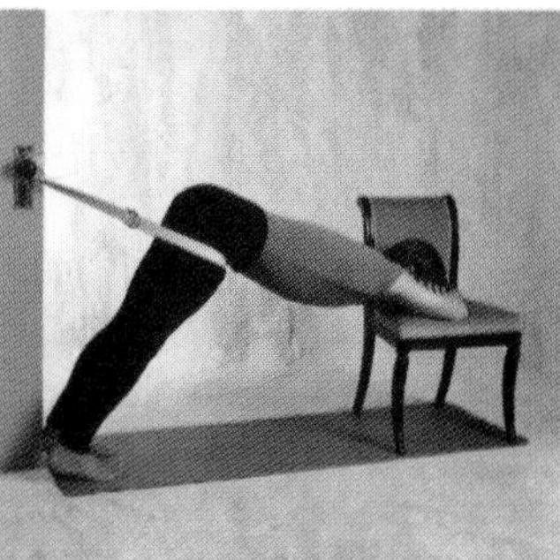

FIGURE 7.2
Hanging Dog Pose, Variation

Setting Up. Spread out your nonskid mat, with the narrow end centered on the edge of the open door. Firmly fasten your belt into a wide loop, and place it around both doorknobs. Step inside the loop, and stand with your back to the door. Hold the belt and walk forward until it presses against your body where the thighs meet the torso.

Bend your knees, lean forward, and put your hands on the floor. Walk your feet back toward the door, and walk your hands forward until your body is in the shape of an inverted V. Let the belt hold the weight of your body. Make sure that the belt pulls evenly against both sides of the door. If your hamstrings are too tight to practice comfortably with your hands on the floor, work with your hands on a chair seat.

Your hands should be approximately 18 inches apart, and so should your feet. In addition, your hands and feet should be a wide distance from each other. Often this pose is practiced with hands and feet too close together. This makes it difficult to feel the wonderful stretch that releases the spine and belly.

Being There. Let your head hang, as you allow the belt to hold your weight. Breathe slowly and evenly, as your back muscles lengthen. As you exhale, move your belly into the pelvis so it forms a concave shape. Relax, confident that you are on your way back to health.

Coming Back. Practice Hanging Dog Pose for 1 minute, gradually increasing to 3 minutes. To come out, bend your knees, walk your hands toward your feet, and stand up. Remain still for a few moments and, with your eyes open, take a few breaths before stepping out of the belt and continuing with your practice.

Benefits. Hanging Dog Pose places the long muscles of the lower back in traction. With the help of gravity, this gentle stretch can relieve tension in the long muscles, as well as in other muscles of the lower back. In addition, Hanging Dog Pose is an inversion, which reverses the normal position that the vertebral structures have in relationship to gravity, thus relieving the habitual postural effects of standing upright.

Cautions

- Remove your socks for this pose.
- Be careful not to lose your balance as you step into or out of the belt loop. If you feel unsteady or uncertain, practice with a stable chair nearby so you can place one hand on it to steady yourself.

Nobody can experience our lives for us.
—Charlotte Joko Beck

Supported Half-Dog Pose

Supported Half-Dog Pose uses a sturdy table to support your torso when you bend forward. This pose gently stretches the long muscles of the back by placing the lower back in traction. As your torso rests on the table, gravity's pull on the back muscles is relieved.

Prop

- sturdy table

Optional Props

- 1 or more single-fold blankets

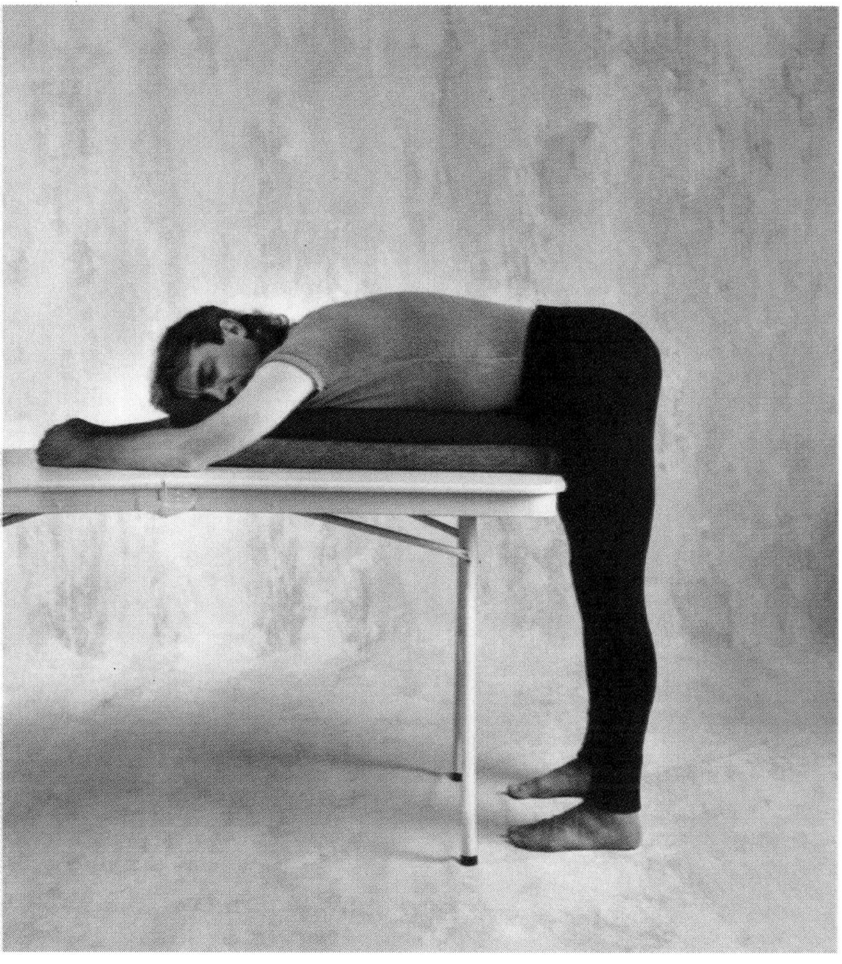

FIGURE 7.3
Supported Half-Dog Pose

Setting Up. Stand in front of the table, feet hip-width apart. Bend forward from where your torso meets your thighs, and rest your torso on the table. Your torso and legs should be at 90 degrees to each other, with your legs straight and feet resting lightly on the floor. If you are not at 90 degrees, come up and stack 1 or more single-fold blankets on top of the table. Come forward again and rest your torso on the blankets. Stretch your arms out in front of you and hold on to the far edge or rest them on the table, or fold your arms and place them on the table.

Rest your forehead either on the table or on your folded arms. You can also turn your head to one side, as long as you spend an equal amount of time with your head turned to the other side.

Being There. Breathe slowly and easily. Let your torso and arms rest completely on the table. Slightly bend your knees, and let the weight of your legs drop toward the floor. Allow your back and neck to lengthen on each exhalation.

Try stretching in this supported position: walk backward a few steps or reach forward with your arms. If you feel any discomfort, skip these stretches for now.

Coming Back. Practice Supported Half-Dog Pose for 2 to 3 minutes. Keeping your knees bent, use your arms to help you come to a standing position. Stand quietly for a few breaths before proceeding to the next pose.

Benefits. Supported Half-Dog Pose stretches the muscles along the spinal column and relieves tightness and stiffness in your lower back.

Cautions

- Remove your socks for this pose.
- Take care not to aggravate your back condition when coming into and out of this pose. If you feel pain as you bend forward and rest on the table, skip the pose for now. Try it again when your back is more cooperative.
- If you experience dizziness when coming into or out of this pose, make sure that you are not holding your breath while moving up or down. If the dizziness recurs the next time you practice this pose, consult your health care professional.
- Do not practice this pose if you are more than three months pregnant.

Perseverance brings success.

—Afro-American Encyclopedia, 1869

Simple Supported Back Bend

Some people with lower back pain prefer rounding the lower back to stretch; others like to arch it. I suggest that you balance your practice and your body by moving your spine in both directions: forward and back. This more accurately reflects the way a healthy back moves during daily activities. Simple Supported Back Bend is a good introduction to back bends if your lower back is sensitive. It's gentle, it improves flexibility, and it's possible for almost anyone.

Props
- bolster
- long-roll blanket

Optional Props
- eyebag
- block
- double-fold blanket
- extra blanket for warmth
- clock or timer

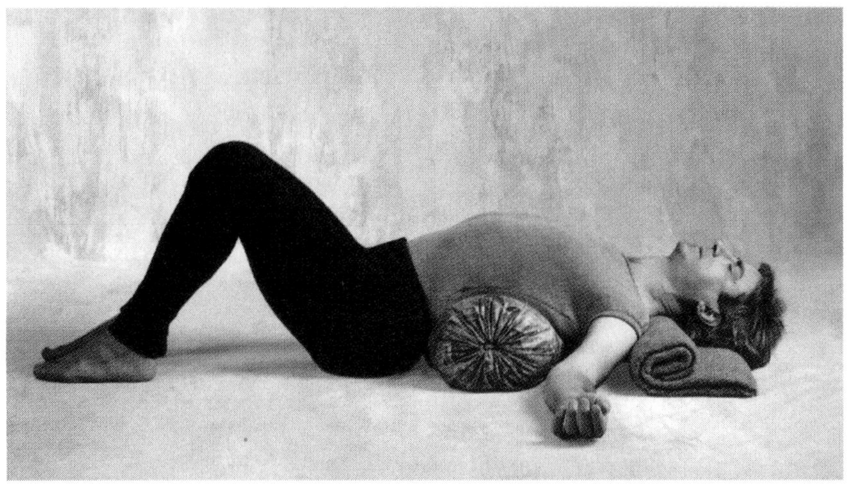

FIGURE 7.4
Simple Supported Back Bend

Setting Up. For the details of setting up this pose, refer to page 31.

Being There. Breathe slowly and evenly. With each inhalation, your front body opens; with each exhalation, your belly and organs soften and your mind quiets. As your relaxation deepens, allow your lower back to soften, as you release all tension.

Coming Back. Practice Simple Supported Back Bend for 1 minute, gradually increasing your time to 4 minutes. To come out, push with your feet and slide toward your head. Rest for a few breaths with your lower back flat on the floor and your legs supported by the bolster. Then roll to the side and sit up slowly.

Benefits. Simple Supported Back Bend is an antidote to slouching, an unhealthy postural habit that rounds the spine and shoulders forward.

Caution
- See page 33 for more advice on this back bend.

Elevated Twist on a Bolster

Props

- bolster
- nonskid mat

Optional Props

- pillow or towel
- extra blanket for warmth
- clock or timer

Elevated Twist on a Bolster is a pleasant way to stretch the external rotator muscles, located deep in the outer hips. It also stretches the muscles at the sides of the rib cage, such as the latissimus dorsi. When these muscle groups are stretched, the function of the lumbo-sacral spine is enhanced.

Short but powerful, the external rotators stabilize the pelvis during movement. They are strengthened by standing on one leg. Some common activities that use the external rotators are serving a tennis ball, pitching a baseball, or kicking a soccer ball. Sometimes these muscles can be overused. Someone who jogs or runs regularly uses the external rotators so frequently and forcefully that the muscles tighten. When they are too tight, the movement of the pelvis over the hip joints is limited. As a result, the rhythm of lower back movements is interrupted. This imbalance can cause muscle strain in the surrounding tissues.

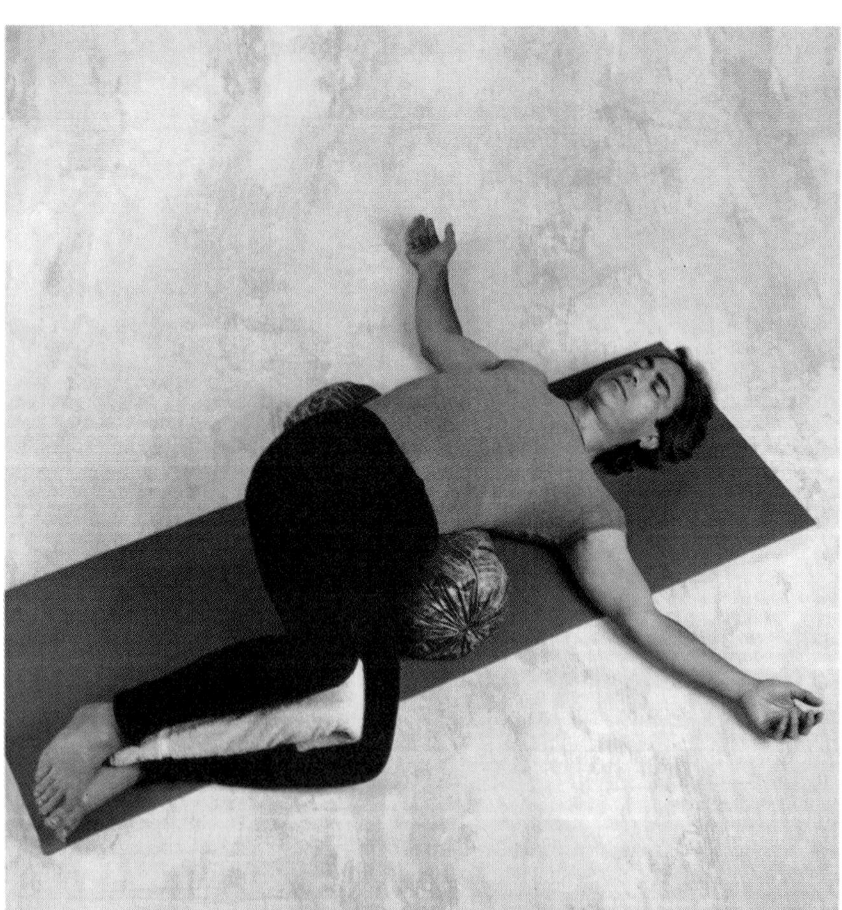

FIGURE 7.5
Elevated Twist on a Bolster

Setting Up. Place a bolster on top of your mat. Sit in the middle of the long side of the bolster. Bend your knees and place your feet on the floor. Slide forward a little and place your hands on the floor behind you. Gently lie back so that your hips rest in the middle of the bolster and your shoulders lightly touch the floor.

The real joy of life is in its play.
—Walter Rauschenbusch

Press your feet into the floor as you slide your hips to the far left side of the bolster. Then move the feet over to align with the hips. Make sure the lowest rib on either side of your back is supported by the bolster. Place your arms on the floor, palms up, so they and your torso form a T shape.

Bring your knees toward your chest, one at a time, until your thighs are at a 90-degree angle to your chest. Keep your knees together as you drop your legs to the right, until they are supported by the bolster. If your external rotators are tight, you will not be able to keep your knees together. Place a pillow or folded towel between your knees to support your upper leg. Let your pelvis roll over too, so you are lying on your right side. If your left shoulder comes up, let it. Stretch out through the left arm and hand.

If you are pain-free, you can add more traction to the twist by straightening both legs once you are in the pose. Remember to keep your knees and feet together. In this position, your thighs remain supported by the bolster, and the lower legs rest on the floor. The body is more twisted when you do this and you are lying more completely on your side. If straightening the legs strains your lower back, keep the knees bent to protect it.

In this pose, the back is slightly arched. Make sure that the chest is not dropped but that you position yourself so your upper back is arched and the chest is open. To arch the chest, lift the breastbone as you press the tailbone down.

Being There. Breathe deeply. Focus on the gentle stretches created by the twist. Balance the stretch between the movement of your knees dropping to the side and the stretch you feel in your shoulder. Enjoy the stretch along the side of your body and your upper chest, in the region of the pectoralis muscles. Feel the stretch in the external rotators of the outer hip. Keeping these muscles flexible is important to the health of your lower back.

Coming Back. Practice Elevated Twist on a Bolster for 1 minute on each side. If you are practicing with straight legs, bend your knees. To come out, roll onto your back and lift your legs one at a time. Lower your feet to the floor and rest for a few breaths.

When you feel ready, repeat the pose to the opposite side. Don't be surprised if the second side is different from the first. Slide off the bolster in the direction of your head and roll to the side. Remain in this position until you feel ready to get up.

Benefits. Elevated Twist on a Bolster is a general tonic for the lower back. It combines the benefits of a twist, which stretches the small muscles of the spine, an inversion, which places the lower back in traction, and a back bend, which helps to release tension on the intervertebral discs. In addition, Elevated Twist on a Bolster stretches the external rotators and the other muscles that hold the pelvis and trunk together, like the latissimus dorsi. It also opens the lungs and diaphragm, which improves respiratory function and enhances general well-being. Finally, this pose stimulates the kidneys.

Cautions

Do not practice this pose:

- if you have a hiatal hernia or heart problems.
- if you are more than three months pregnant.
- if you are menstruating.

What you will do matters.
All you need is to do it.
—JUDY GRAHN

Supported Child's Pose

When adequately supported, Supported Child's Pose is just about everyone's favorite, especially if your lower back aches from prolonged standing or sitting. Do not skip this pose because it looks too simple. It is quite effective, especially when sequenced after the previous two poses, which arched the spine. Back bends are often new movements for many people. Bending forward, or flexing, the lumbar spine in Supported Child's Pose provides a counterbalancing movement.

Prop

- bolster

Optional Props

- 1 or more single-fold blankets
- 2 towels
- sandbag
- long-roll blanket
- extra blanket for warmth
- clock or timer

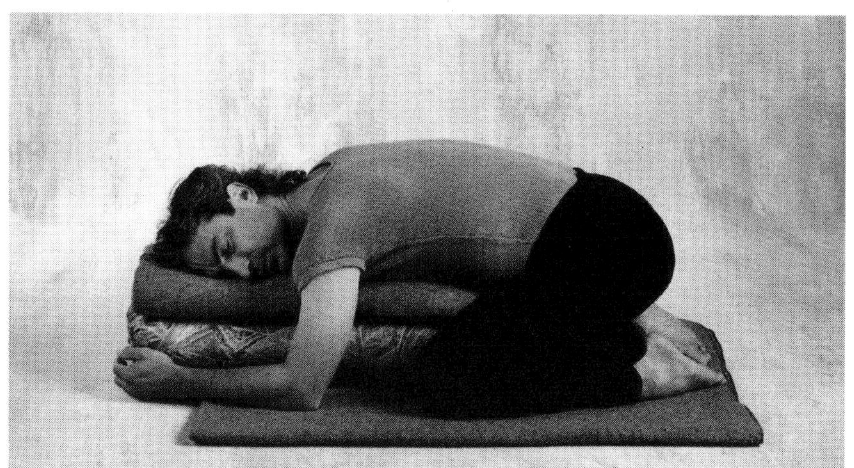

FIGURE 7.6
Supported Child's Pose

Setting Up. See page 58 for the details of setting up this pose.

Being There. Take several slow breaths. As you do, allow yourself to drop down and receive the support of the bolster. Continue to breathe and let your shoulders move away from the ears.

Let your tailbone move toward the floor and your entire lower back area soften and spread. Take a long slow inhalation, as you release all tension from your lower back. Let this relaxation seep into the entire pelvic area, both through the spinal structures and into the abdomen.

Coming Back. Practice Supported Child's Pose for 1 to 3 minutes. Be sure that you spend equal time with your head turned in each direction. Open your eyes. Reach back with one hand, and slide the sandbag off your back and to one side. Place your palms on the floor, under your shoulders. Press your hands into the floor, inhale, and sit up slowly onto your heels. Rest for a moment and come to a kneeling position. Immediately place one foot on the floor, place your hands on that thigh, and inhale deeply as you come to a standing position.

Benefits. Supported Child's Pose gently stretches the lower back, relieves shoulder tension, and quiets the mind.

Caution

- See page 59 for more advice on this pose.

Basic Relaxation Pose with Legs on a Chair

Props

- chair
- single-fold blanket
- eyebag

Optional Props

- sandbag
- 1 or more single-fold blankets
- extra blanket for warmth
- clock or timer

This series concludes with Basic Relaxation Pose. In this variation, the legs rest on a chair seat, and a sandbag is placed on the lower abdomen. When you first place weight on the abdomen, your breathing may feel constricted. As layers of tension release and your abdomen accepts the weight, you will notice that the sandbag feels lighter and your breathing easier. As the abdomen relaxes, so does the lower back.

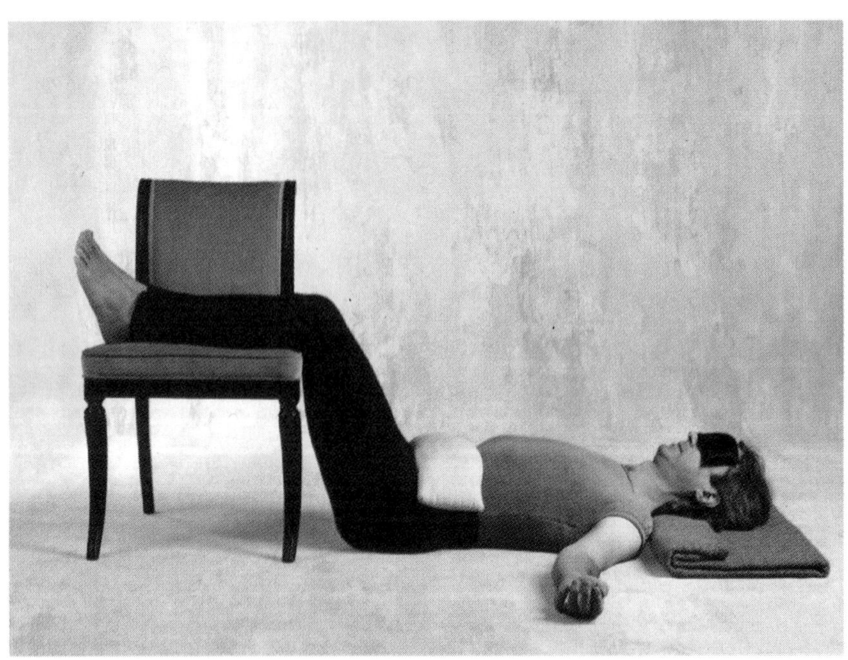

FIGURE 7.7
Basic Relaxation Pose with Legs on a Chair

Setting Up. Begin by sitting on the floor, with the chair in front of you and your standard-fold blanket behind you. Use the strength and support of your arms to help you lie back. Place your lower legs on the chair seat, so your knees and hips are bent. If you need an extra blanket for warmth, cover your legs with an unfolded one.

If your lower legs do not rest easily on the chair seat, it may be that your thighs are not long enough to reach it. If so, bring the knees toward the chest, roll gently onto your side, and sit up using your arms. You can elevate your torso in relationship to the chair by lying on one or more single-fold blankets.

Next, roll the long edge of your standard-fold blanket slightly to support the gentle curve of your neck. Adjust the prop placement under your head and neck so you are comfortable. Your chin should be slightly lower than your forehead.

When you are comfortably settled, place a sandbag on your lower abdomen. If you are using an extra blanket for warmth, pull it up to cover your torso and arms. Allow your upper eyelids to soften down toward the lower lids as your eyes close. Cover your eyes with an eyebag.

Rest with your arms out to the sides, so your upper arms do not touch the sides of your rib cage. Most people practice with the palms turned up, but if this is not comfortable, turn them down and let the elbows relax.

Being There. Read the detailed instructions under Being There on page 26, if you are not yet familiar with being in Basic Relaxation Pose.

In addition, allow your lower back to sink downward and any tension to melt away and be absorbed by the floor. Feel a release in the muscles of your lower back, and send this part of your body permission to let go and be pain-free.

When you feel ready, begin the Centering Breath: a long, slow, gentle inhalation, followed by an exhalation of equal length, followed by several cycles of normal breathing. (See pages 24 and 26 for complete instructions.) Repeat this process for up to 10 breaths. Be sure to leave some time for normal breathing before coming out of the pose.

Coming Back. If you are practicing with a sandbag on your abdomen, come out of the pose when it feels as if the weight is gone, or nearly gone. If you are not using a sandbag, practice this variation of Basic Relaxation Pose for 15 to 20 minutes. To come out, remove the eyebag and then slide the sandbag to one side off your body. Rest here for several breaths. Then roll to the side and use your arms to help you sit up.

What you see is what you get.
—FLIP WILSON

Benefits. This variation of Basic Relaxation Pose relaxes the muscles and organs of the abdomen, as well as the muscles of the lower back, and refreshes the legs.

Cautions

- If you are more than three months pregnant, practice Side-Lying Relaxation Pose (see chapter 13).
- Do not use the sandbag if you are menstruating.
- Take care as you come out of the pose. Walk around the room a few times to try out your relaxed back. When you resume your normal activities, try to avoid bending and twisting at the same time.

The quality of our practice is always reflected in the quality of our life.
—CHARLOTTE JOKO BECK

PRACTICE SUMMARY

The length of your practice may depend on time available and how you feel. Here is a summary of the Down in the Back series, followed by suggestions on using poses from the series to practice for shorter periods of time.

25 to 35 Minutes

POSE	TIME
Hanging Dog Pose	2 to 3 minutes
Supported Half-Dog Pose	2 minutes
Simple Supported Back Bend	2 to 4 minutes
Elevated Twist on a Bolster	2 to 3 minutes
Supported Child's Pose	2 to 3 minutes
Basic Relaxation Pose with Legs on a Chair	15 to 20 minutes

5 Minutes

POSE	TIME
Basic Relaxation Pose with Legs on a Chair	5 minutes

15 Minutes

POSE	TIME
Hanging Dog Pose	2 minutes
Supported Child's Pose	3 minutes
Basic Relaxation Pose with Legs on a Chair	10 minutes

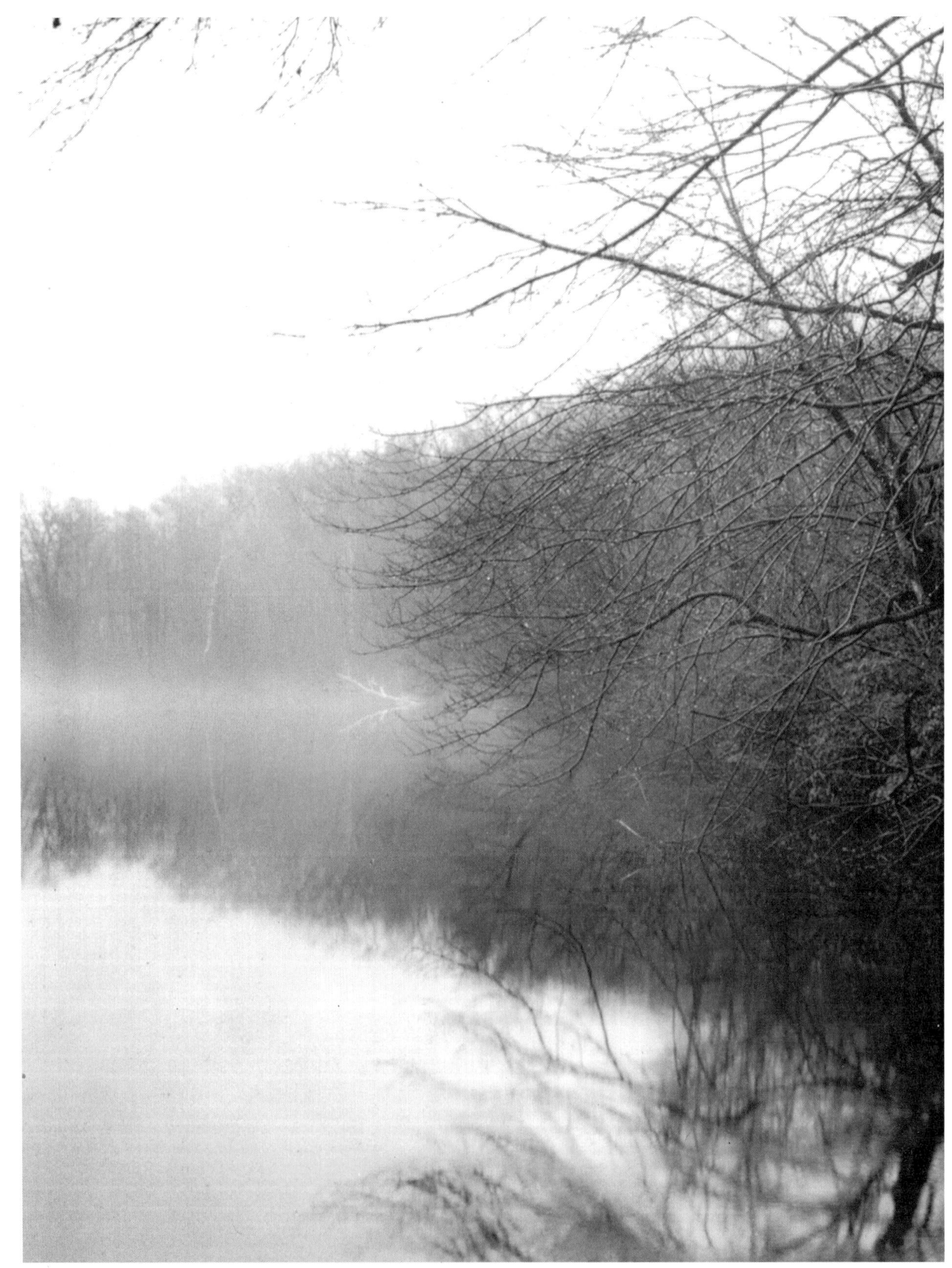

CHAPTER EIGHT

A PAIN IN THE NECK

Poses for Headaches

HEADACHES, which always seem to come at exactly the wrong time, are caused by a variety of things, including hunger, monosodium glutamate (MSG) in food, caffeine, hangovers, cigarette smoke, tight glasses, dental or sinus problems, cold temperatures of air or food, or watching television or reading for long hours. Tension headaches, muscle contraction headaches, and migraine headaches are the types that cause most sufferers to seek advice.[1]

Just as their name implies, tension headaches are caused by tension, made worse if you are feeling depressed or anxious. They usually last all day and are frequently characterized by a tightening sensation or general pressure around the head. Often these headaches can be relieved by relaxing, without use of any drug or therapy.

Muscle contraction headaches are primarily due to poor standing and sitting postures that are held for hours at a time. The dynamics are simple: When you sit or stand for a long time, the natural curves of the spine are stressed because they are usually held out of alignment. In response to this misalignment, almost continual contraction occurs in the muscles of the upper back, shoulders, and neck. This tension is actually your body's attempt to hold itself upright in a difficult, distorted position. The muscles of the neck and shoulders become knotted and fatigued, as they try to resist gravity.

Migraine headaches differ in that they are caused by vascular, or blood vessel, changes in the brain, affecting blood circulation. If you suspect your headache might be a migraine, or if you experience incapacitating headaches accompanied by nausea and digestive or visual disturbances, or any headache that is excessive or constant, see your health care professional. The poses in this chapter are not intended for migraine headaches.

Restorative yoga can relieve the discomfort caused by tension as well as muscular contraction headaches. These poses can also help you create the habit of being relaxed, a habit that may prevent future headaches.

The Pain in the Neck Series

This series consists of four restorative yoga poses: three modified inversions to relax your legs, back, and shoulders, and a variation of Basic Relaxation Pose in which the legs rest on a bolster to facilitate overall body relaxation. These poses address not only the tension of the headache itself, but the tension created in the body by reacting to the headache.

There is nothing permanent except change.
—HERACLITUS

The series takes from 30 to 60 minutes. As always, I encourage you to be realistic about what is possible. Give yourself as much time to practice these poses as you can. Your neck and shoulder tension patterns have developed over time, so it may take some time to undo them. Using poses from the full series, shorter practice sessions are suggested in the Practice Summary at the end of the chapter.

In addition to practicing restorative yoga poses, I recommend two things. First, approach your headaches with an attitude of prevention. Good body mechanics are important. Attention to posture can often ease the tension in the neck and shoulders. Remember, poor sitting and standing posture not only affects your neck and shoulders but also your breathing, digestion, and elimination. (See chapters 16 and 17 for practical suggestions for improving sitting and standing postures.) Second, consider that while practicing this series is useful, its effects are even more sustainable if you can stay relaxed throughout the day. Practice the shorter routines for home and office from chapter 6.

Wrapping the Head

What is unique about the Pain in the Neck series is that you wrap your head with an elastic bandage, a technique developed by Iyengar. When properly positioned, the elastic bandage places pressure on the frontalis muscle of the forehead, as well as on the temples and sinuses. It also screens out light, often a contributing irritant to headaches. An elastic bandage is especially handy to have with you if you get headaches while traveling. It is one yoga prop that tucks easily into your suitcase.

The results of a study published in the journal *Headache* (January 1993) concur with Iyengar's empirical findings. Using a simple elastic and Velcro device called the Headache Band, which maintains pressure on points that provide relief, twenty-five patients reported positive effects in sixty out of sixty-nine headaches tested.[2]

How to Use the Elastic Bandage

You can use an elastic bandage for all the poses in the Pain in the Neck series. The elastic bandage is wrapped mainly around your forehead but also is intended to lightly cover your eyes. Do not wrap your head in a way that places pressure on the eyes themselves, and remove your glasses or contact lenses first.

Unroll 6 to 8 inches of the bandage. Begin to wrap it around your head, starting at the base of your skull. Hold the rolled portion in one

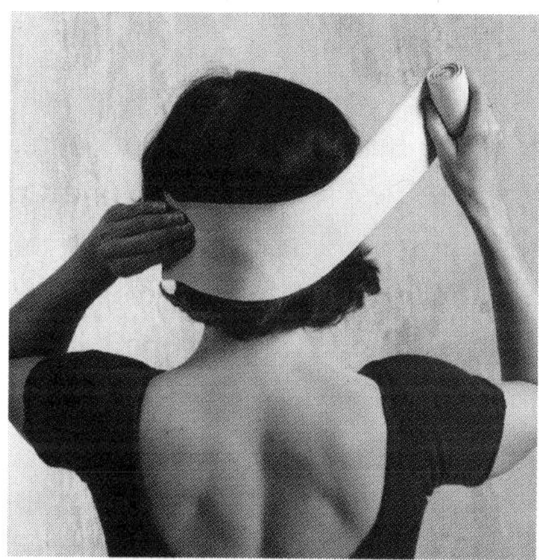

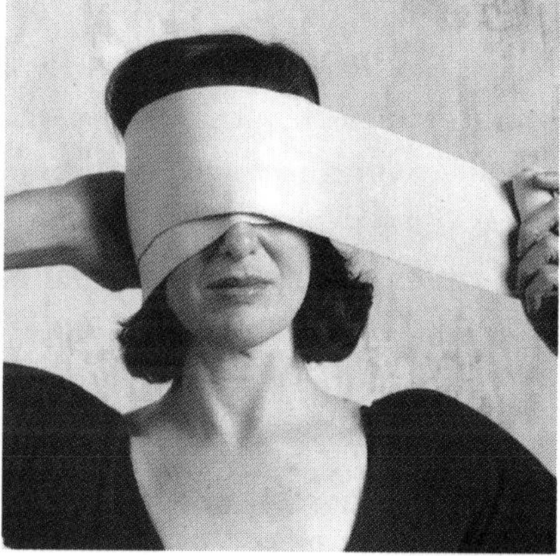

FIGURE 8.1
Starting the Head Wrap

FIGURE 8.2
Continuing the Head Wrap

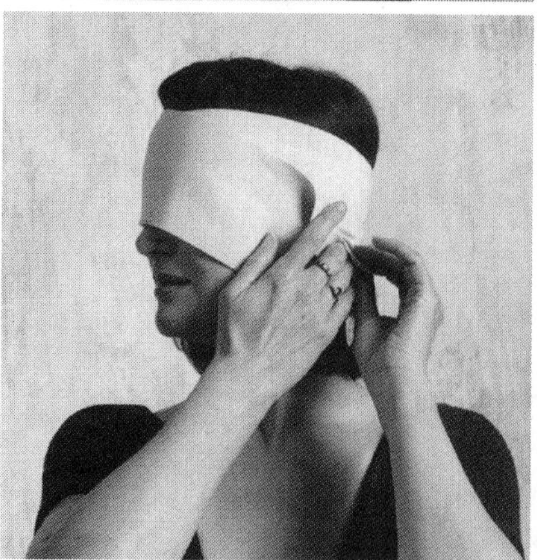

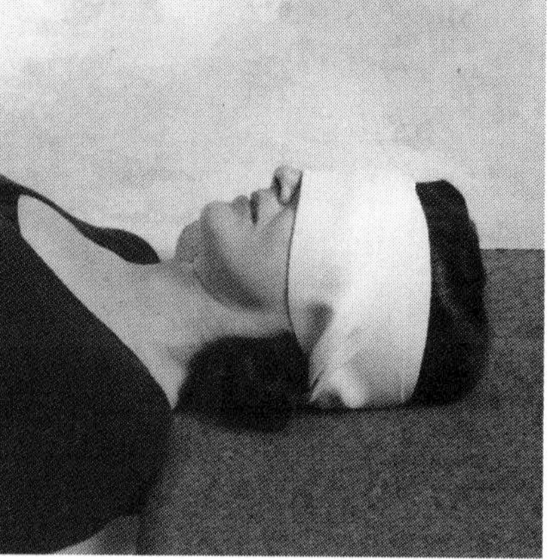

FIGURE 8.3
Tucking in the Head Wrap

FIGURE 8.4
Practicing with the Head Wrap

hand, and gently hold the loose end against your head, just behind your ear, with your other hand. Close your eyes. Slowly but surely wrap the bandage around your head: around the base of your skull, over your ear, and crossing over one eye by directing the bandage up. On the next round, cross over the other eye by directing the bandage downward. Continue to wrap the bandage around your head, and then tuck in the end wherever convenient. Avoid tucking it in at the back of your head, where it might make an uncomfortable lump when you lie down during practice.

In between poses, fold up the front of the wrap away from the eyes so you can see to set up the next pose. To remove the head wrap at the end of the series, unwind it slowly so that the gentle pressure on your head is released gradually.

I recommend that you practice putting the bandage on and taking it off several times before combining its use with the poses. I also recommend that you practice each pose a few times without the bandage, so you develop the familiarity and confidence to do so literally with your eyes closed.

Alternatives to the Elastic Bandage

If you like the feeling of having your head wrapped, you can use the bandage in all the poses in the series. If the head wrap feels confining or makes your headache worse, take it off. Here are three alternatives to try in the supine poses. Variation 1 uses a towel, books, and an eyebag; variation 2 uses books, a sandbag, and an eyebag; variation 3 uses an eyebag only. All three variations relieve tension in the frontalis, the muscle that draws your eyebrows upward.

Variation 1. Place a towel so it rests just above your brows, on your forehead. Let the rest of the towel drape over the top and sides of your head and onto the floor. Place two or more books on the towel on either side of your head, close to your ears, and on the towel above your head.

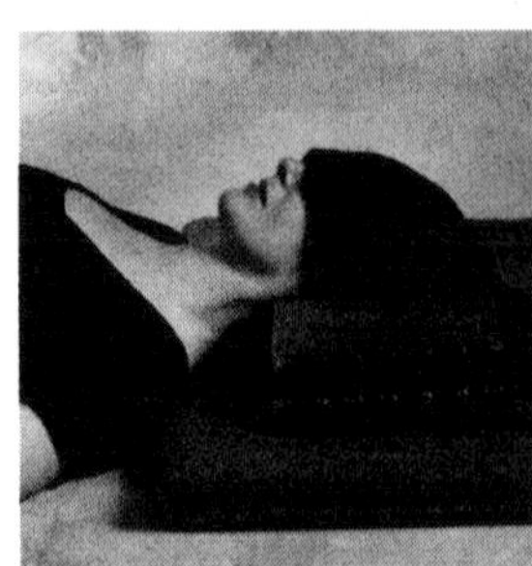

FIGURE 8.5
Head Wrap, Variation 1

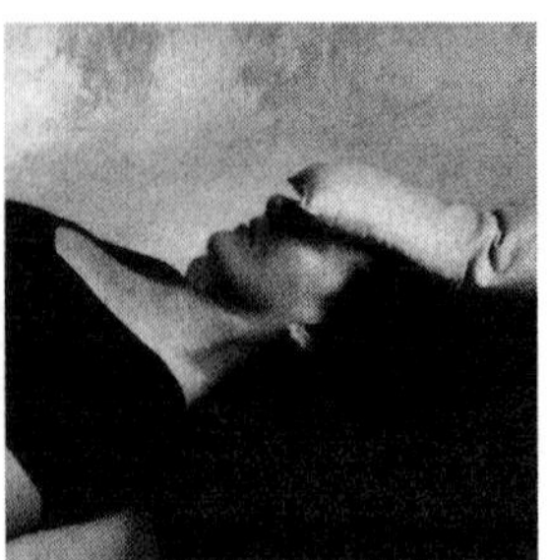

FIGURE 8.6
Head Wrap, Variation 2

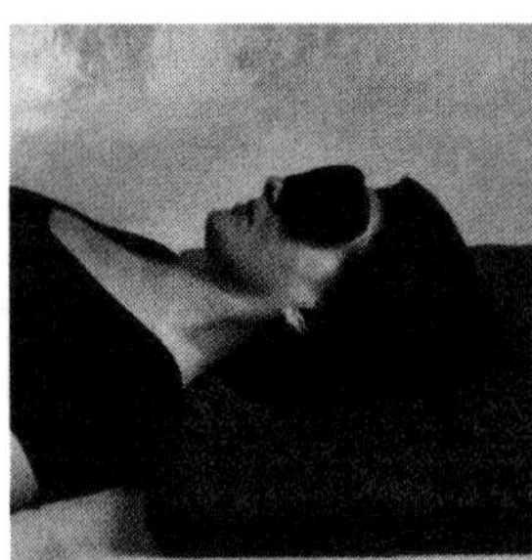

FIGURE 8.7
Head Wrap, Variation 3

The weight of the books will help to press the towel against your forehead. You can also place an eyebag over your eyes.

Variation 2. Place the books on the floor, close to the top of your head. Carefully lay a sandbag on top of the books and bring approximately one-third of it forward to rest on your forehead. You can also place an eyebag on your eyes.

To love oneself is the beginning of a lifelong romance.
—Oscar Wilde

Variation 3. Place the eyebag either on your eyes or on your forehead. Whichever alternative you use, first read through the instructions for each pose to determine where your head will be positioned. Then place your props so you can reach them easily, without disturbing your position in the pose.

Neck and Shoulder Care

In addition to restorative yoga, be sure to take care of your neck and shoulders during the day and while you sleep. These few strategies may help prevent those nagging headaches.

- Don't slump in your chair. See chapter 17 for some tips on sitting well.
- Don't hunch one shoulder when talking on the telephone. Alternate the hand you use to hold the phone, or try a headset.
- Don't drop your head forward as you read or work at the computer. This strains the muscles at the back of the neck. Use a stand to hold your reading material at eye level, and position your computer screen so it is just below eye level.
- Don't carry everything on one shoulder. Lessen your load—you probably don't need to carry it all anyway. Alternate your carrying shoulder or consider using a backpack for even distribution of weight. If you do use a backpack, make sure it rides high and comfortably near your shoulders. If it hangs near your waist, it will cause back discomfort.
- Don't stick your neck out when driving. Keep your ears over your shoulders.

How restful is your sleep? Your neck should be supported, so the spine is in good alignment and the muscles of the neck and shoulders aren't strained. Get a good pillow, or sleep with a rolled-up towel under your neck along with a pillow.

Supported Half-Dog Pose

Prop

- table

Optional Props

- 1 or more single-fold blankets
- elastic bandage
- clock or timer

You can practice Supported Half-Dog Pose in more situations than many of the other restorative poses because it doesn't require many props and you don't lie on the floor. Try it at your kitchen table, at your desk or lunch table at work, or on a picnic table.

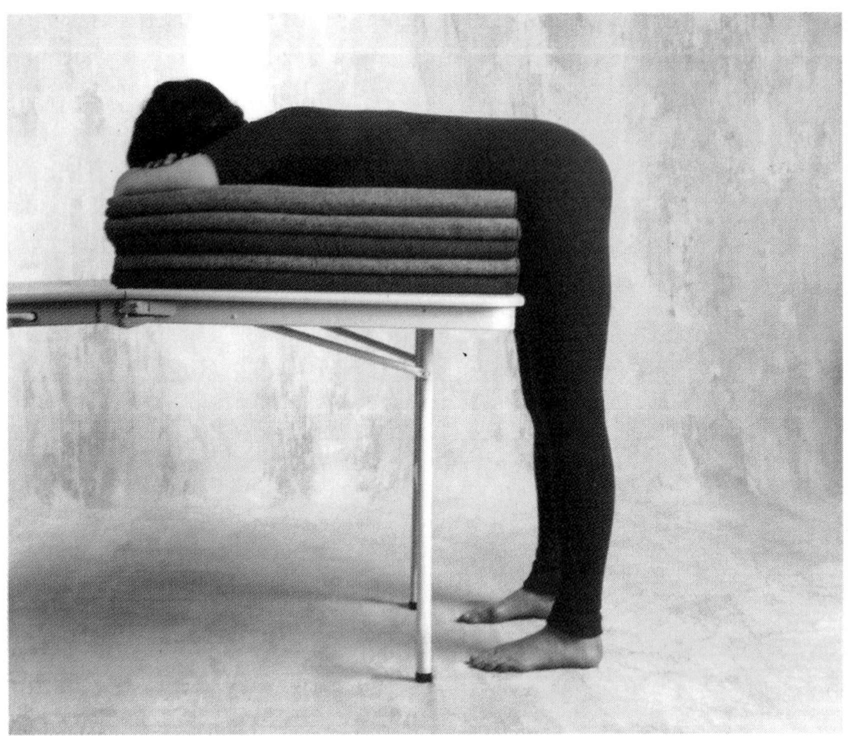

FIGURE 8.8
Supported Half-Dog Pose

Setting Up. Refer to page 75 for a complete description of setting up Supported Half-Dog Pose. If you are using a head wrap, put it on before coming forward.

Being There. Try stretching in this supported position. You can walk backward a few steps if it feels good; you can also reach your arms forward if it feels good. Easy stretching may relieve the tension in your upper back, shoulders, and neck. Be careful not to overdo it; do not practice this part of the pose if it makes your headache worse.

Coming Back. Practice Supported Half-Dog Pose for up to 5 minutes. Bend your knees and use your arms to help you come to a standing position. If you're using the elastic bandage, fold the front of the wrap up away from the eyes so you can see to set up the next pose. Slowly open your eyes. Stand quietly for a few breaths before proceeding to the next pose.

Benefits. Supported Half-Dog Pose gently stretches the long muscles of the lower back and rests the muscles of the upper back, neck, and shoulders. Aided by the table, the muscles of the back are placed in gentle traction.

Caution

- See page 76 for more advice on this pose.

Supported Bridge Pose

Supported Bridge Pose stretches the muscles at the back and sides of the neck. This stretch can relieve an existing headache and prevent future ones. We create neck tension by the postural habit of carrying the head in front of the torso. Positioning your head even 1 inch forward of a vertical position can greatly increase muscle tension in the back of the neck. Along with this tension comes the gradual shortening of the muscles and other connective tissue, such as ligaments and tendons around the joints.

Props

- 2 bolsters

Optional Props

- 2 or more single-fold blankets
- elastic bandage or alternative
- towel
- extra blanket for warmth
- clock or timer

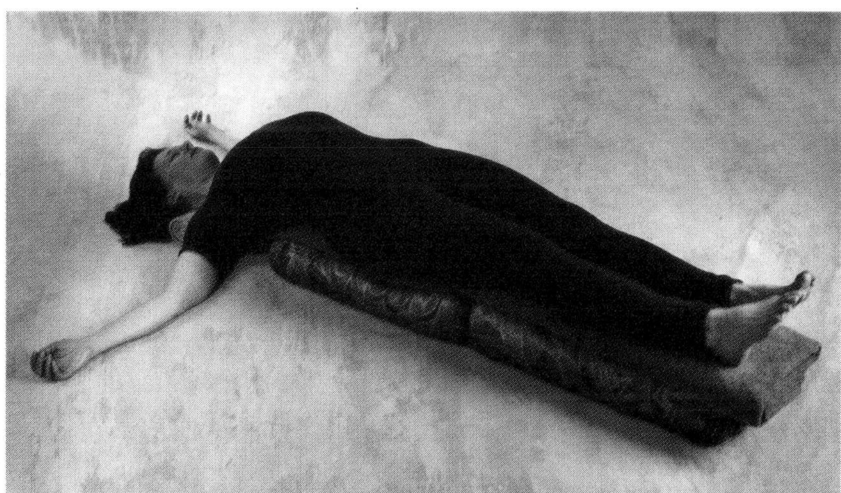

FIGURE 8.9
Supported Bridge Pose

Setting Up. Refer to page 39 for details on setting up Supported Bridge Pose.

Once you have your props ready, sit down, straddling the bolsters, and move slightly nearer to the end behind you. If you are using a head wrap, reposition it to cover your eyes.

Use the support of your arms to help you lie down. Carefully slide off the end toward your head, so your shoulders touch the floor and you face the ceiling. Adjust the position of the rolled towel under your neck so you are completely comfortable.

If you are not using a head wrap but would like to use one of the alternatives, put it on now. Place your arms out to the side at a comfortable angle.

Being There. To enhance your relaxation, let your eyeballs turn downward, and let the forehead feel broad and flat.

Swallow and let the jaw and tongue relax. Allow your neck muscles to feel long and released. Notice the gentle arch of the neck, spanning from the base of the shoulders to the base of the skull. Release all tension at the base of the skull.

Gently bring your attention to your breathing. Feel the lateral movement of your lungs and ribs with each inhalation and exhalation. Rest, poised between the energy of thought drawing inward and the energy of the body opening and expanding.

Coming Back. Practice Supported Bridge Pose for 5 to 15 minutes. If you are using a head wrap alternative, remove it now. To come out, slide off the bolsters in the direction of your head. Rest your lower legs on the bolster, with your back on the floor. Stay for a few minutes. Roll to one side. Press down with your hands and sit up slowly. If you're using the elastic bandage, fold up the front of the wrap away from the eyes so you can see to set up the next pose. Slowly open your eyes.

Benefits. Supported Bridge Pose stretches the muscles of the neck, opens the chest, and encourages breathing. Holding the breath in response to stress creates more stress and contributes to a headache.

Caution

- See page 40 for more advice on this inverted pose.

We have to try to cure our faults
by attention and not by will.
—Simone Weil

Elevated Legs-Up-the-Wall Pose

Elevated Legs-Up-the-Wall Pose is one of the most effective ways to relieve the all-over body ache that often accompanies a headache. In this restorative yoga pose, the legs rest, the chest opens, the brain cools, and whole body releases tension.

Props

- bolster
- single-fold blanket

Optional Props

- elastic bandage or alternative
- double-fold blanket
- 1 or more single-fold blankets
- standard-fold blanket
- towel
- extra blanket for warmth
- clock or timer

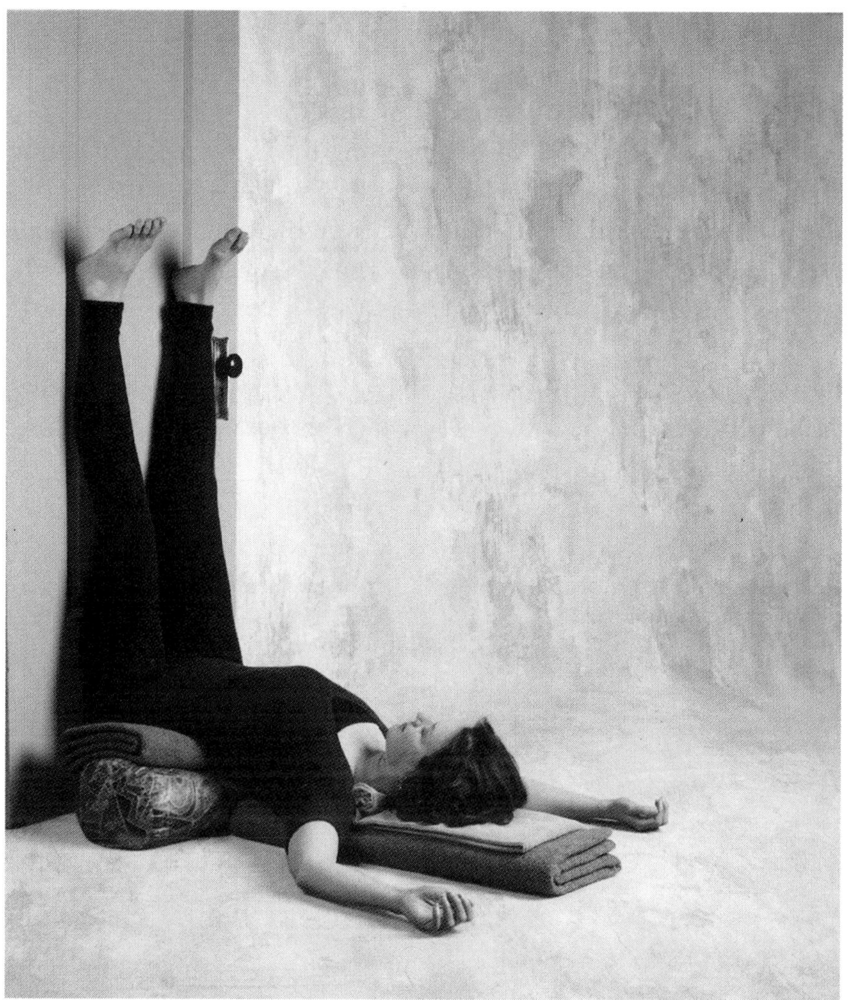

FIGURE 8.10
Elevated Legs-Up-the-Wall Pose

Setting Up. Follow the instructions in page 41 to set up this pose. If you are using a head wrap, reposition it to cover your eyes. If you are using an alternative to the head wrap, put it on once you are settled.

Being There. Remain present to your breath and bodily sensations. As you become aware of each sensation, mentally describe it—for example, pressure, throbbing, aching, or whatever fits. Don't get lost in thinking about each sensation or judging yourself because the headache is not going away. Just note and briefly describe each sensation.

As you open yourself to your own experience, the pain may become worse. Continue to open to the sensations, and after the initial increase in pain, the headache will begin to subside.

Coming Back. Practice Elevated Legs-Up-the-Wall Pose for 10 to 15 minutes. If you are using an alternative to the head wrap, remove it now. Lie still for several breaths before opening your eyes.

Bend your knees, press your feet on the wall, and lift your pelvis up a little. Push the bolster toward the wall with your hands, and slide your body away from the wall by pressing with your feet. Lie on the floor a few moments, with your lower legs supported by the bolster. Then roll to the side and get up slowly. If you're using the elastic bandage, fold up the front of the wrap away from the eyes so you can see to set up the next pose. Slowly open your eyes.

Benefits. Elevated Legs-Up-the-Wall Pose stretches the back and sides of the neck. It also opens the chest, which encourages deep breathing and relaxation.

Caution

- See page 43 for more advice on this inverted pose.

There is a salve for every sore.

—Afro-American Encyclopedia, 1869

Basic Relaxation Pose with Bolster

Tension headaches are a common result of living under chronic stress. While specific restorative poses stretch and release the neck, back, and shoulders, Basic Relaxation Pose is the most important pose for headache relief. Not only does it relax your neck and shoulders, but it has systemic circulatory benefits that may even relieve migraines.

Props

- standard-fold blanket
- bolster

Optional Props

- elastic bandage or alternative
- extra blanket for warmth
- clock or timer

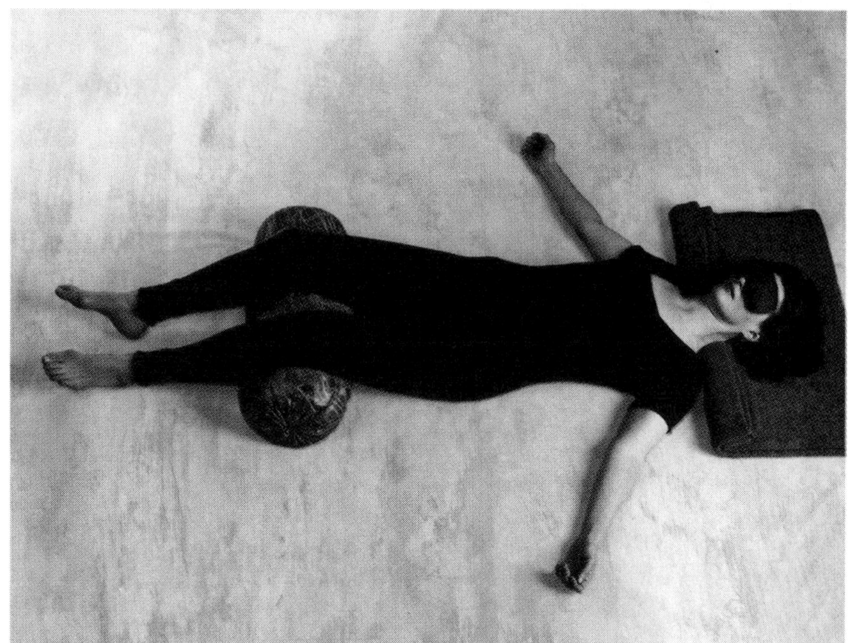

FIGURE 8.11
Basic Relaxation Pose with Bolster

Setting Up. Refer to Setting Up, page 25, for complete instructions on Basic Relaxation Pose. As usual in this pose, position a standard-fold blanket for your head and neck to rest on. Place a bolster under your knees. If you have a tendency to get cold, cover yourself with an unfolded blanket. If you are using a head wrap, reposition it to cover your eyes. Then use the strength and support of your arms to help you lie back. If you are using a head wrap alternative, put it on after you lie down.

Being There. Imagine that your brain is getting smaller as it moves away from the skull. Relax your eyeballs and forehead. Let your lower back sink downward, and let any tension melt away and be absorbed by the floor. Feel a release in the muscles of your lower back.

Let your attention rest on the easy rise and fall of the abdomen with each breath. When you feel ready, begin your practice of the Centering

Breath as described on page 26. Remember, never force the breath. Repeat the Centering Breath for up to 10 rounds. Be sure to leave some time for normal breathing before coming out of the pose. Allow yourself to rest in the here and now.

Coming Back. Practice Basic Relaxation Pose with Bolster for 5 to 25 minutes. If you are using an alternative to the head wrap, remove it now. To come out of the pose, inhale and as you exhale, draw one knee toward your chest, then the other, and in a natural rhythm roll to one side.

Rest on your side for a few breaths. To sit up, press the floor with the elbow of your lower arm and the palm of the upper hand. If you are using the head wrap, remove it now. Sit quietly for several breaths before standing up and resuming your normal activities.

Benefits. Basic Relaxation Pose with Bolster releases muscular tension, lowers blood pressure, and slows the heart rate. In addition, it reduces fatigue from lack of sleep due to a headache.

Caution

- If you are more than three months pregnant, practice Side-Lying Relaxation Pose in chapter 13 instead.

Simplicity is the most difficult thing to secure in this world; it is the last limit of experience and the last effort of genius.
—George Sand

PRACTICE SUMMARY

The length of your practice may depend on time available and how you feel. Here is a summary of the Pain in the Neck series, along with some suggestions for using these poses in shorter practice periods.

30 to 60 Minutes

POSE	TIME
Supported Half-Dog Pose	5 minutes
Supported Bridge Pose	5 to 15 minutes
Elevated Legs-Up-the-Wall Pose	10 to 15 minutes
Basic Relaxation Pose with Bolster	10 to 25 minutes

10 Minutes

POSE	TIME
Basic Relaxation Pose with Bolster	10 minutes

20 Minutes

POSE	TIME
Elevated Legs-Up-the-Wall Pose	5 minutes
Supported Bridge Pose	5 minutes
Basic Relaxation Pose with Bolster	10 minutes

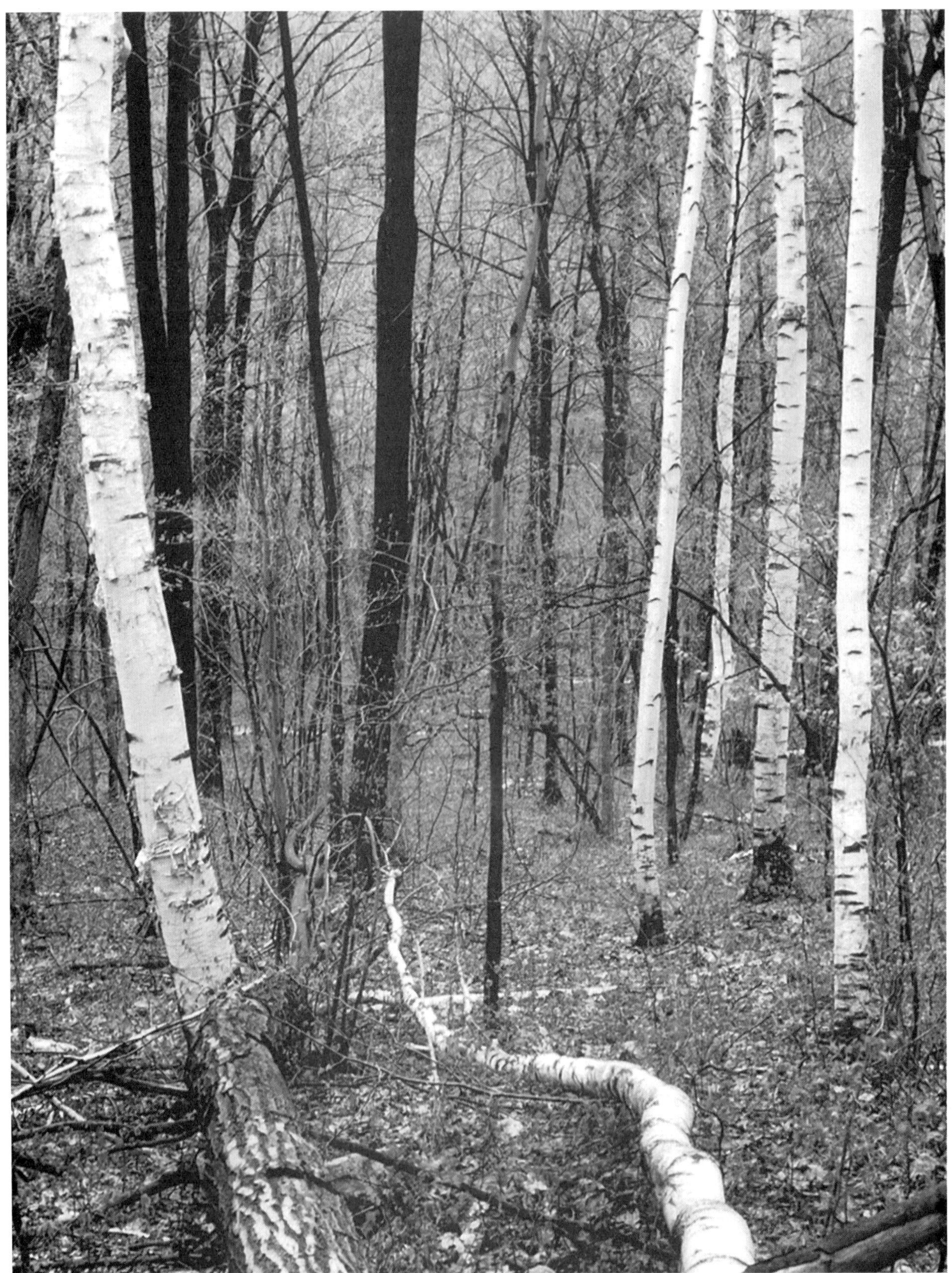

CHAPTER NINE

ELUSIVE DREAMS

Poses for Insomnia

Do you spend the wee hours of the morning tossing and turning? Punching your pillow into a more comfortable shape? Throwing off your covers one minute and pulling them up the next? Checking the clock, hoping that morning is not far off? If so, then you already know that nothing is more tiring than trying to fall asleep. And you are not alone. Each year millions of people consult their physicians regarding sleep problems.

Insomnia, or chronic sleeplessness, often stems from stress. When overstimulated by stress, we become agitated, which makes it difficult to fall asleep. As a result of being deprived of a good night's sleep, we become unbalanced and more vulnerable to the stress that caused the problem to begin with. This vicious cycle is compounded when the sleeplessness continues from night to night.

Insomnia was one reason I turned to yoga. At the time, I was looking for a nondrug alternative to help me bypass the habitual one to two hours it took me to fall asleep. I realized that my inability to relax body and mind directly affected my sleep. Through yoga I learned new habits; you can, too.

The Elusive Dreams Series

What is mind? It doesn't matter.
What is matter? Never mind.
—**Anonymous**

The Elusive Dreams series is designed to help soothe your senses before retiring, so that you fall asleep with ease. It consists of six restorative yoga poses, beginning with two supported reclining poses to start the relaxation process. These are followed by a supported back bend to deepen your relaxation, and a modified inversion to reduce your overall fatigue. Next is a supported seated pose to quiet your mind. The series concludes with a variation of Basic Relaxation Pose in which the legs are slightly elevated to relax your lower back, abdomen, and legs.

I recommend that you include the 40- to 60-minute Elusive Dreams series in your nightly routine before bed. If you do not have time for the entire series, see the Practice Summary at the end of this chapter for two shorter practice sessions using poses from the series.

If you wake up in the middle of the night and cannot fall back to sleep, get out of bed. It is important that you associate your bed with sleep and not with insomnia.[1] Once out of bed, practice some or all of the poses from the Elusive Dreams series. Even if you don't fall asleep, the more you relax, the more successful you will be in breaking the cycle of insomnia.

As you relax your body with the Elusive Dreams series, you will also learn to relax your mind. In yoga there is a practice called *pratyahara.* A Sanskrit term, it means "the conscious withdrawal of energy from the senses." Often misunderstood as shutting oneself away from the external world, pratyahara more accurately means that while sensory input is registered in the mind, this input does not disturb the mind. Ideally this is what happens during conscious relaxation: you learn to remain aware of your bodily sensations and your thoughts without being swept away by them. This is an important skill to master, especially if you are being kept awake by ruminations on the past, the future, or the what-ifs of life.

As you practice the Elusive Dreams series, notice how your thoughts come and go. Neither push your thoughts away nor become attached to them. Instead, just notice the continual cycle of thoughts arising and falling away, understanding that they are not who you are, any more than the sounds that emanate from a piano are the piano.

Wrapping the Head

We will use the elastic bandage to enhance relaxation, as in the previous chapter. See page 89 for instructions on wrapping your head and using alternatives to the elastic bandage. You can use an elastic bandage for all of the poses in the Elusive Dreams series. This chapter includes specific instructions for the use of props in each pose.

Other Simple Ways to Help You Sleep

In addition to the Elusive Dreams series, I recommend that you actually plan to get a good night's sleep. The following strategies will help.

- Practice Basic Relaxation Pose for 5 to 10 minutes one or two times during the day in addition to the Elusive Dreams series in the evening.
- Get a massage in the late afternoon or early evening to help you wind down after the day.
- Take a warm bath before your Elusive Dreams practice each evening.
- Drink a cup of warm milk just before bedtime.
- Avoid overstimulating activities after 7 P.M., such as exercise, watching television, listening to loud music, or eating a big meal.

::: PRACTICE

Supported Reclining Pose

Supported Reclining Pose can help you reprogram your nervous system and undo the habit of insomnia. This pose resembles relaxing in a chaise lounge, so put down your worries for the next 10 minutes and imagine you're resting on a warm, white-sand beach of a tropical island, trusting that all is well.

Props

- bolster
- 1 or more single-fold blankets
- 1 or more standard-fold blankets
- 3 long-roll blankets

Optional Props

- elastic bandage or eyebag
- extra blanket for warmth
- clock or timer

Setting Up. Place your bolster on the floor, with a single-fold blanket on one end to support your head. Next, roll a standard-fold blanket around at least one long-roll blanket, with the size determined by your comfort. Position this large roll near the bolster so you can reach it easily. Also place a long-roll blanket on either side of the bolster for use under each elbow and forearm. Experiment with which height works best for you. This added support will enhance your relaxation; it is recommended for those with carpal tunnel syndrome or with whiplash or other neck problems.

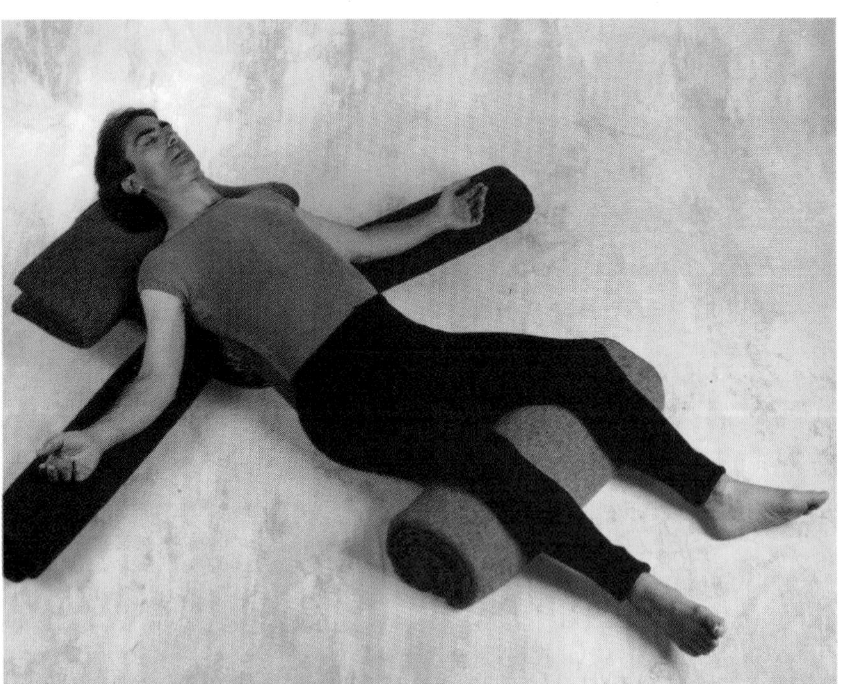

FIGURE 9.1
Supported Reclining Pose

Sit in front of the short side of your bolster with it touching your tailbone. Bend your knees and place the large blanket roll under them. If you are using a head wrap, put it on now. Lean back and rest your torso on the bolster and your head on the single-fold blanket. Let your legs and feet roll out and your heels rest on the floor. If you are using an eyebag, put it on now.

Place your forearms on the props, palms up. If you prefer your palms turned down, make sure the curve of each palm is supported by the blanket.

If you have any back discomfort, sit up as described in Coming Back. Experiment with adding 1 or more single-fold blankets to your props: sit on one; place another on the bolster. Add another single- or standard-fold blanket to support your head. Lie down again, reposition yourself on the props, and reassess your comfort.

Being There. Settle into the props, allowing your forehead to feel broad under the head wrap. Swallow to relax your throat and jaw. Let the lower jaw fall away from the upper jaw, and let your cheeks drop into the hollow just below the cheekbones.

Take several long, slow breaths. As you exhale, make an audible sigh as you allow your belly to drop into the pelvis. Do this several times. Allow all tension to drain away. When your body feels soft and diffuse, take a few more long, slow, easy breaths.

As you relax, you may experience more physical comfort but more mental agitation. Relaxing is like peeling an onion. As you remove the top layer, the next layer reveals itself. Allow space for your mental agitation—not pushing it away, not judging it. Just notice what arises in your body and in your mind, as layer after layer of tension reveals itself and releases.

Coming Back. Practice Supported Reclining Pose for 10 minutes or longer, depending on your comfort. It is virtually impossible to overdo this pose. If you are using an eyebag, remove it, keeping your eyes closed to adjust to the light before opening them. Bend your knees and use your feet to push away the large blanket roll. Roll to one side and lie there for several breaths before sitting up. If you are using the head wrap, fold the front of the wrap up away from the eyes so you can see to set up the next pose. Slowly open your eyes.

Benefits. Supported Reclining Pose helps those with lung congestion by reducing the tendency to cough, relieves tension between the shoulder blades, and is beneficial for the kidneys. Practicing with the head wrap increases the depth of relaxation.

Cautions

- In Supported Reclining Pose, it is important that your head and chest are higher than your belly. It is also important that your chest does not collapse, but lifts.
- If you feel discomfort in your lower back, come out of the pose immediately. Adjust the props so you can be pain-free. If this is not possible, skip the pose for now. If you are fine in the pose but feel discomfort after you practice, keep the props the same but practice for less time the next time.

If you leave your mind as it is,
it will become calm.
This mind is called big mind.
—Shunryu Suzuki

Supported Bound-Angle Pose

Props

- bolster
- 4 long-roll blankets
- double-fold blanket
- belt or sandbag

Optional Props

- elastic bandage or eyebag
- single-fold blanket
- extra blanket for warmth
- clock or timer

Although it might seem like an extreme route to relaxation, sensory deprivation (or flotation) tanks operate on the premise that it is impossible to relax and sustain relaxation if the nervous system is continually bombarded by stimuli. You can experience the same soothing effect of reduced sensory input and replace overstimulation with warmth, darkness, and quiet by regular practice of Supported Bound-Angle Pose. Enhanced by the support of the bolster, blankets, and head wrap, this pose can help you achieve a deep level of relaxation.

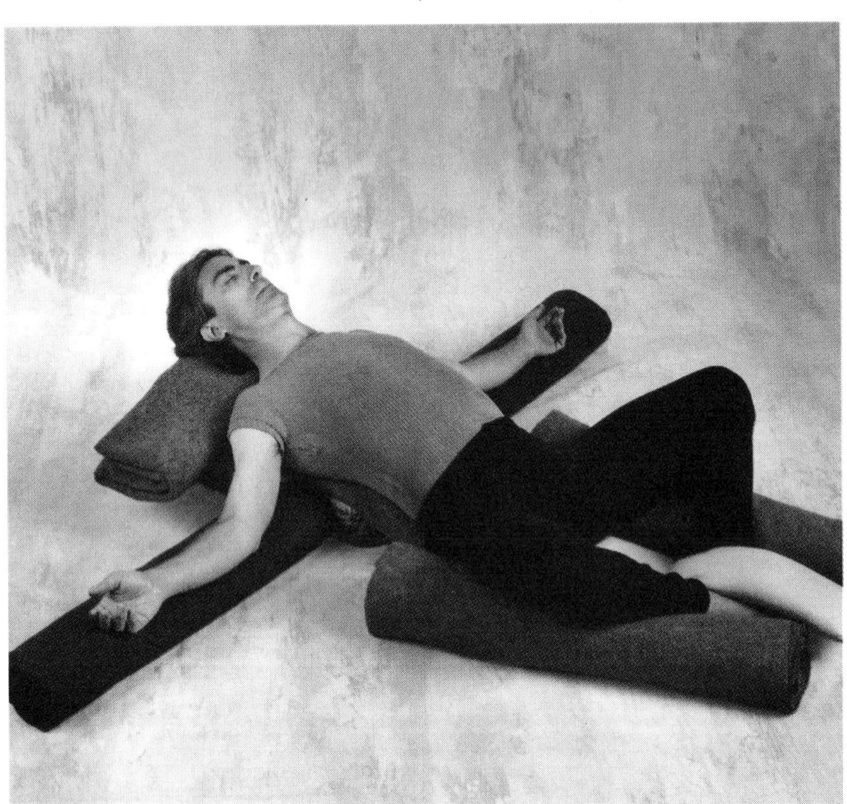

FIGURE 9.2
Supported Bound-Angle Pose

Setting Up. Follow the instructions on page 34 to set up this pose. If you are using a head wrap, reposition it to cover your eyes after securing your feet in place, soles together. If you use an eyebag, put it on after you lie down.

Being There. As you settle in, let the props do the work. Don't try to relax; imagine that you have left your worries and tendency to try too hard at the door. Rest easy.

When you feel ready, begin the Centering Breath: a slow, gentle inhalation, followed by a slow, gentle exhalation, followed by several normal cycles of breath, until you feel refreshed and ready to begin the Centering Breath again. (See pages 24 and 26 for a complete discussion of the Centering Breath.) As you breathe, trust that you can learn good sleep habits; as you exhale, release all tension and worry. Be sure to leave some time for normal breathing before coming out of the pose.

Coming Back. Practice Supported Bound-Angle Pose for 10 minutes, longer if you are comfortable, shorter if that is what you can do for today. After relaxing so deeply, let the outside world come slowly into your awareness. Take in the sounds around you; pay attention to the sensations of your body.

If you are using an eyebag, remove it and slowly open your eyes. To come up, press down with your arms and sit up slowly. If you are using the head wrap, fold the front of the wrap up away from the eyes so you can see to undo the belt or remove the sandbag from your feet. Slowly stretch your legs out in front of you to release any tension in the knees. Quietly move to the next pose.

Benefits. Supported Bound-Angle Pose reduces fatigue, which is particularly important if you are caught in the insomnia cycle. In addition, the pose enhances breathing and relieves headaches. It is useful for those with digestive problems, especially indigestion, because of the pose's positive effect on the liver and stomach. It is beneficial for women during menstruation (see chapter 12) and menopause (see chapter 14).

Caution

- See pages 35 and 36 for advice on this pose.

The greatest ideas,
the most profound thoughts,
and the most beautiful poetry
are born from the womb
of silence.
—William A. Ward

Mountain Brook Pose

Props

- bolster
- 2 single-fold blankets
- long-roll blanket

Optional Props

- standard-fold blanket
- elastic bandage or alternative
- extra blanket for warmth
- clock or timer

It is revealing to notice how often you hold your breath during your daily activities. Most people do it dozens of times a day! Holding your breath is both a response to and cause of stress and fatigue. Mountain Brook Pose is an excellent way to support the chest so you can breathe more fully and smoothly.

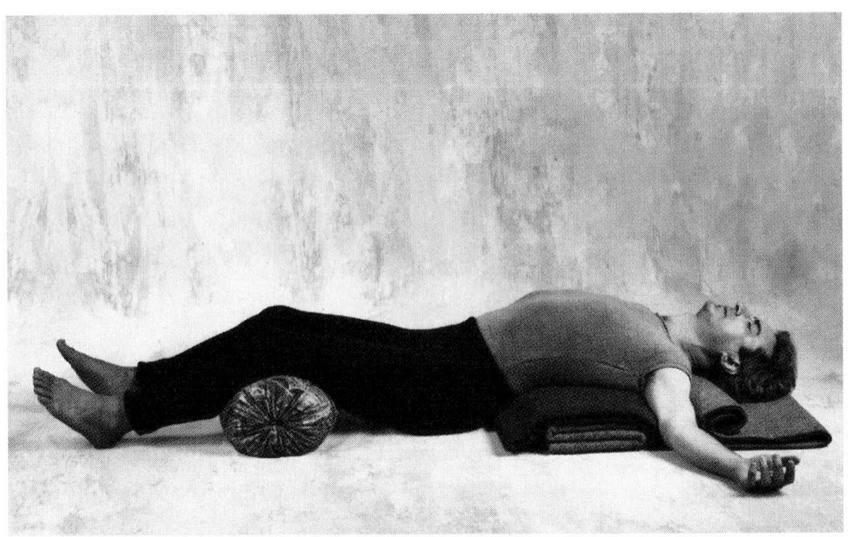

FIGURE 9.3
Mountain Brook Pose

Setting Up. Follow the instructions on page 36 to set up this pose. If you are using a head wrap, reposition it to cover your eyes before you lie back on the props. Put alternatives to the wrap in place after lying back.

Being There. With eyes closed, relax the muscles behind your ears, down through the jaw, and all the way to your chin. Allow your lips to part slightly. Let your tongue rest easily in your mouth. Swallow to relax any tension in your throat. Give up your unspoken words, especially those you tell yourself about how to fall asleep and why you don't fall asleep.

As you continue to breathe and feel the support of the props, gently bring your attention to the open position of your arms and to your heart. Imagine that you are free of all resistance that keeps you from falling asleep easily.

With each exhalation, allow your belly to drop toward your spine. Imagine that your body is softening and spreading, and that you are free of all obstacles to falling asleep. As you continue to relax, breathe normally, enjoying the freedom you feel in your throat, heart, and belly.

Coming Back. Practice Mountain Brook Pose for 4 minutes. If you are very comfortable or are an experienced yoga student, stay for as long as 15 minutes. If you have a stiff back, start with 1 minute and gradually increase your time in the pose.

If you are using a head wrap alternative, remove it and gently lift your head with your hands. Then use your hands to help you slide off the props toward your head. Let your legs rest over the bolster. Lie on the floor for a few minutes before rolling to one side and getting up. If you are using the head wrap, fold the front of the wrap up away from the eyes so you can see to set up the next pose.

Benefits. Mountain Brook Pose helps to alleviate the fatigue and agitation that can accompany insomnia. It counteracts a slumped sitting posture and opens the chest to help you breathe fully.

Caution

- See page 38 for more advice on this pose.

It takes solitude, under the stars, for us to be reminded of our eternal origin and our far destiny.
—**Archibald Rutledge**

Elevated Legs-Up-the-Wall Pose

Props

- bolster
- single-fold blanket

Optional Props

- elastic bandage or alternative
- double-fold blanket
- 1 or more single-fold blankets
- standard-fold blanket
- extra blanket for warmth
- clock or timer

Consider the rhythmic movements of a wave. It alternately crashes onto the shore and then slides back into a seamless ocean. Its movement is like our lives: we spend considerable time advancing into activity and other times receding into quiet reflection. When this rhythm is disrupted, usually it is because we have sacrificed the quiet time to the demands of activity. Practice Elevated Legs-Up-the-Wall Pose to restore this balance, which is particularly important if your overactivity has pushed you into insomnia.

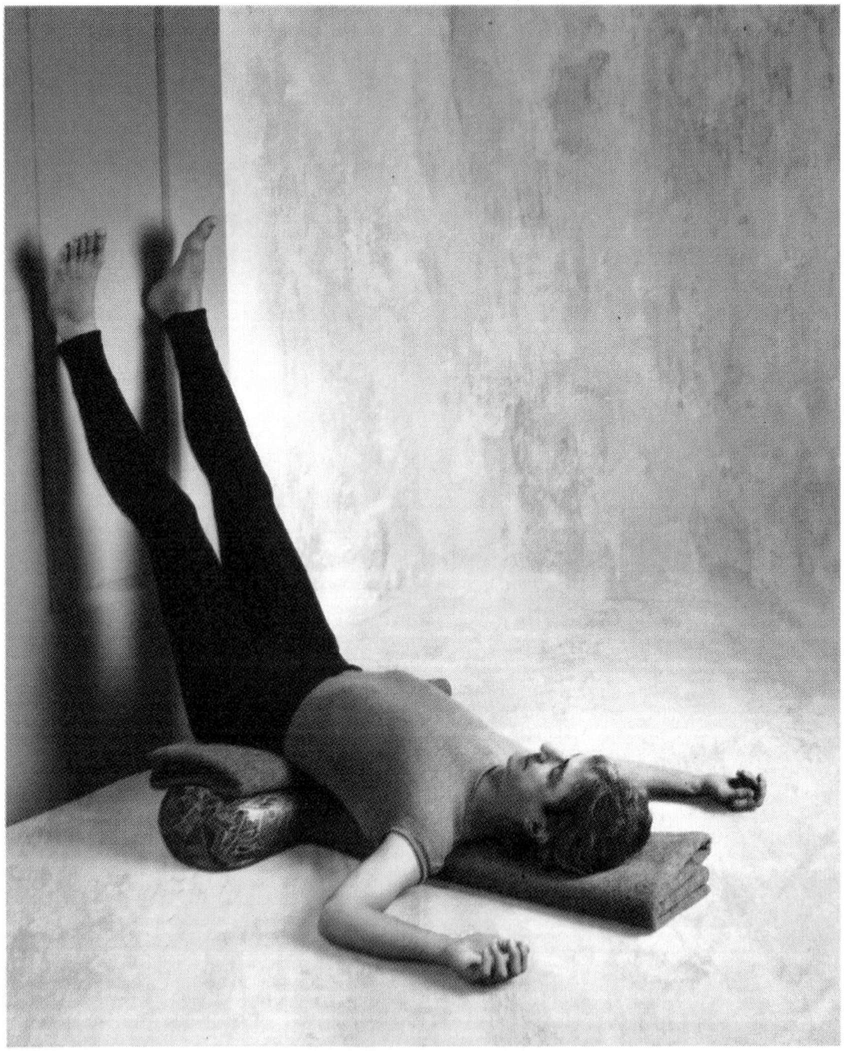

FIGURE 9.4
Elevated Legs-Up-the-Wall Pose

Setting Up. Follow the instructions on page 41 to set up this pose. If you are using a head wrap, reposition it to cover your eyes. If it is difficult to get into the pose with the head wrap in place, cover your eyes once you are in the pose or try a head wrap alternative instead. Put the latter in place after lying back.

Being There. Rest, trusting that you are completely supported by the bolster, the floor, and the wall. Allow yourself the important task of doing nothing. Breathe gently. On each inhalation, imagine that a refreshing breath washes over you. On each exhalation, imagine that, just as a wave slides back to the vast ocean darkness, you are slipping into the silence of the present moment. Accept yourself as you are, trusting that you can relax and sleep.

Coming Back. Practice Elevated Legs-Up-the-Wall Pose for 10 minutes. If you are using a head wrap alternative, take it off now. To come out, bend your knees, press your feet on the wall, and lift your pelvis slightly. Push the bolster toward the wall with your hands, and slide your body away from the wall by pressing with your feet. Lie on the floor for a few moments, with your lower legs supported by the bolster. Roll to the side and get up slowly. If you are using the head wrap, fold the front of the wrap up away from the eyes so you can see to set up the next pose.

Benefits. Elevated Legs-Up-the-Wall Pose relieves the systemic effects of insomnia. It reduces fatigue, quiets the mind, and refreshes the heart and lungs. In addition, it is beneficial for varicose veins and for those who retain water and whose legs swell easily and those who stand for long periods.

Caution

- See page 43 for advice on this inverted pose.

When you hold the breath,
you hold the soul.
—B.K.S. Iyengar

Supported Seated-Angle Pose

Prop

- bolster

Optional Props

- chair
- 1 or more single-fold blankets
- towel
- elastic bandage or alternative
- extra blanket for warmth
- clock or timer

A forward bend, Supported Seated-Angle Pose is cooling and calming to all systems of the body. As you bend forward and rest on the support, it is easier to release tension in the back muscles. The pressure on the forehead releases contraction in the frontalis, a muscle that biofeedback trainers maintain is a reliable indicator of general stress.

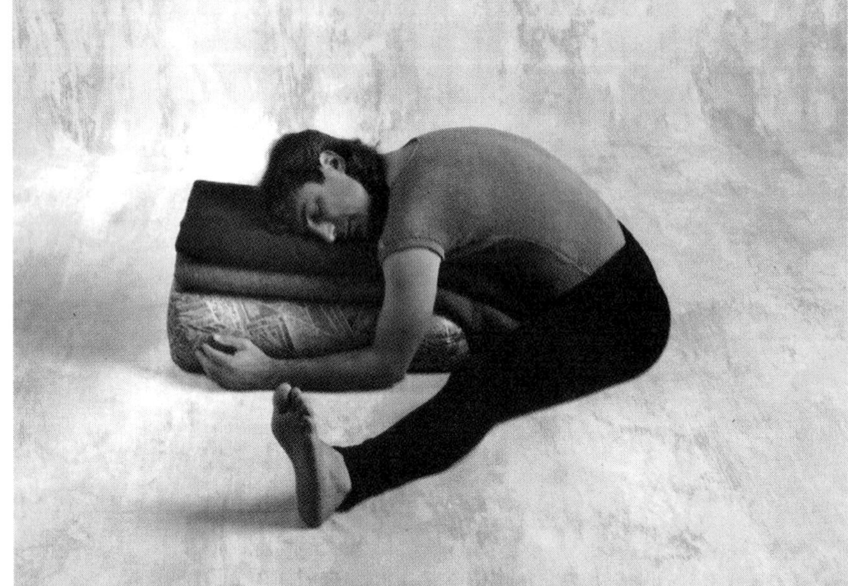

FIGURE 9.5 Supported Seated-Angle Pose

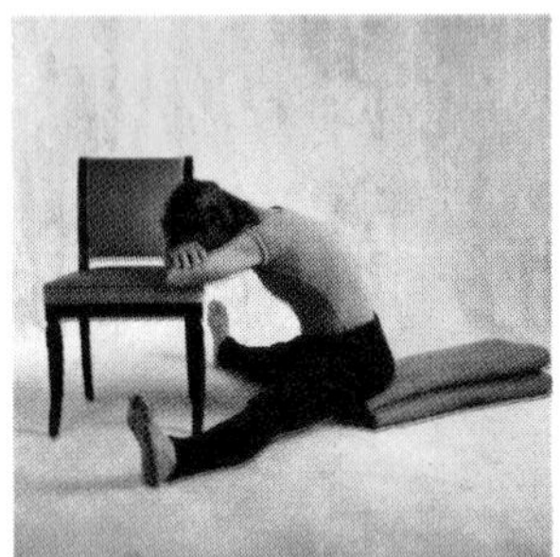

FIGURE 9.6 Supported Seated-Angle Pose, Variation

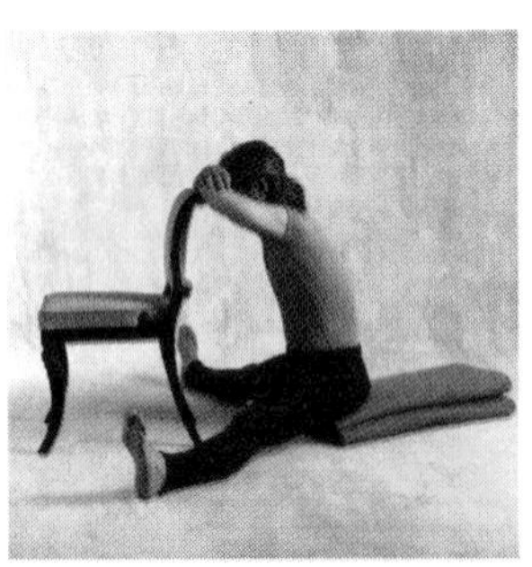

FIGURE 9.7 Supported Seated-Angle Pose, Variation

Setting Up. Follow the instructions on page 46 to set up this pose. If you are using a head wrap, reposition it to cover your eyes before you lean forward.

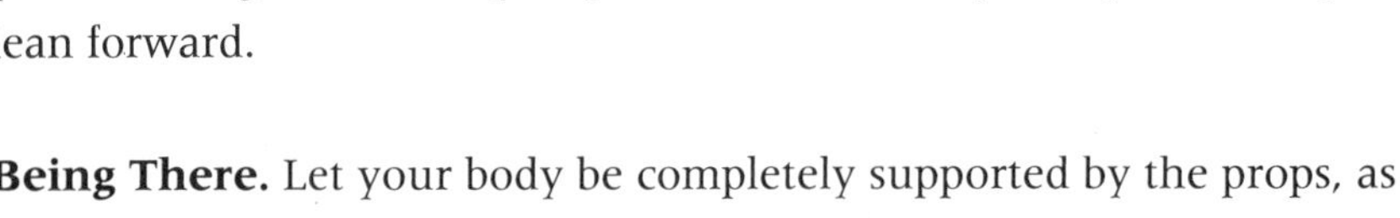

Being There. Let your body be completely supported by the props, as you rest and breathe with eyes closed. Feel the sensations of your body as the external world fades away. There are no demands on you now, no need to be perfect—not even in the pose.

As you continue to breathe, allow your chest to receive the breath and your belly to soften. If your attention is pulled to the chatter in your head, gently guide your attention back to your bodily sensations and the breath. This practice helps you let go of the cares of the day as you fall asleep.

Coming Back. Practice Supported Seated-Angle Pose for 1 to 5 minutes. Come up slowly. If you are using the head wrap, fold the front of the wrap up away from the eyes so you can see to set up the next pose. Lean back on your hands for several breaths to relieve your back.

Benefits. Supported Seated-Angle Pose quiets the organs of digestion and elimination, such as the stomach, intestines, and liver. In addition, this pose balances the squeezing effect on the spine and kidneys of the previous two back bends and opens the lower back area.

Caution

- See page 48 for advice on this pose.

Basic Relaxation Pose with Bolster

Props

- standard-fold blanket
- bolster

Optional Props

- elastic bandage or alternative
- extra blanket for warmth
- clock or timer

The Elusive Dreams series concludes with a variation of Basic Relaxation Pose. People with insomnia are plagued with the worry that they won't be able to fall asleep, which increases as night approaches. If you were fortunate enough to fall asleep but wake up at 2:00 A.M., the anxiety about not being able to fall back to sleep takes over. What to do? Short-circuit the worry by comforting yourself with this pose. Even if you don't fall asleep, you will benefit from relaxing. But most important, you will have replaced the negative thoughts that spiral into hours of discomfort with a positive action of self-care.

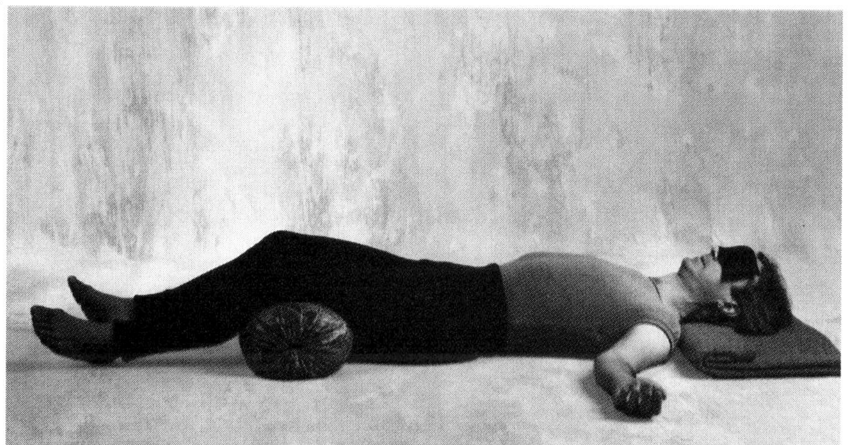

FIGURE 9.8
Basic Relaxation Pose with Bolster

Setting Up. Refer to Setting Up, page 25, for complete instructions on Basic Relaxation Pose. As usual in this pose, position a standard-fold blanket for your head and neck to rest on. Place a bolster under your knees. If you have a tendency to get cold, cover yourself with an unfolded blanket. If you are using the head wrap, reposition it to cover your eyes. Then use the strength and support of your arms to help you lie back. If you are using a head wrap alternative, put it on after you lie down.

Everybody gets so much information all day long that they lose their common sense.
—Gertrude Stein

Being There. Refer to page 26 for guidance in physical relaxation. Let your attention settle on the easy rise and fall of the abdomen with each breath. When you feel ready, begin the Centering Breath (see pages 24 and 26). Practice this for 10 cycles. Rest until you feel completely refreshed.

Coming Back. Practice Basic Relaxation Pose for 5 to 20 minutes. If you are using an alternative to the head wrap, remove it now. To come out of the pose, draw your knees to your chest, one at a time. Roll to one side. Rest in this position for a few breaths. To sit up, press the floor with the elbow of your lower arm and the palm of the hand of your upper arm. If you are using the head wrap, remove it now. Sit quietly until you are ready to resume your normal activities.

Benefits. Basic Relaxation Pose with Bolster reduces the fatigue, stress, and anxiety that accompany insomnia. In addition, it lowers blood pressure and heart rate, and enhances immune system function. Most important, it will teach you how to relax, which is the key to falling asleep easily.

Caution

- If you are more than three months pregnant, practice Side-Lying Relaxation Pose (see chapter 13).

PRACTICE SUMMARY

The length of your practice may depend on time available. Here is a summary of the Elusive Dreams series, along with some suggestions on using poses from the series in shorter practice periods.

40 to 60 Minutes

POSE	TIME
Supported Reclining Pose	10 minutes
Supported Bound-Angle Pose	10 minutes
Mountain Brook Pose	4 minutes
Elevated Legs-Up-the-Wall Pose	10 minutes
Supported Seated-Angle Pose	1 to 6 minutes
Basic Relaxation Pose with Bolster	5 to 20 minutes

10 Minutes

POSE	TIME
Basic Relaxation Pose with Bolster	10 minutes

20 Minutes

POSE	TIME
Elevated Legs-Up-the-Wall Pose	10 minutes
Basic Relaxation Pose with Bolster	10 minutes

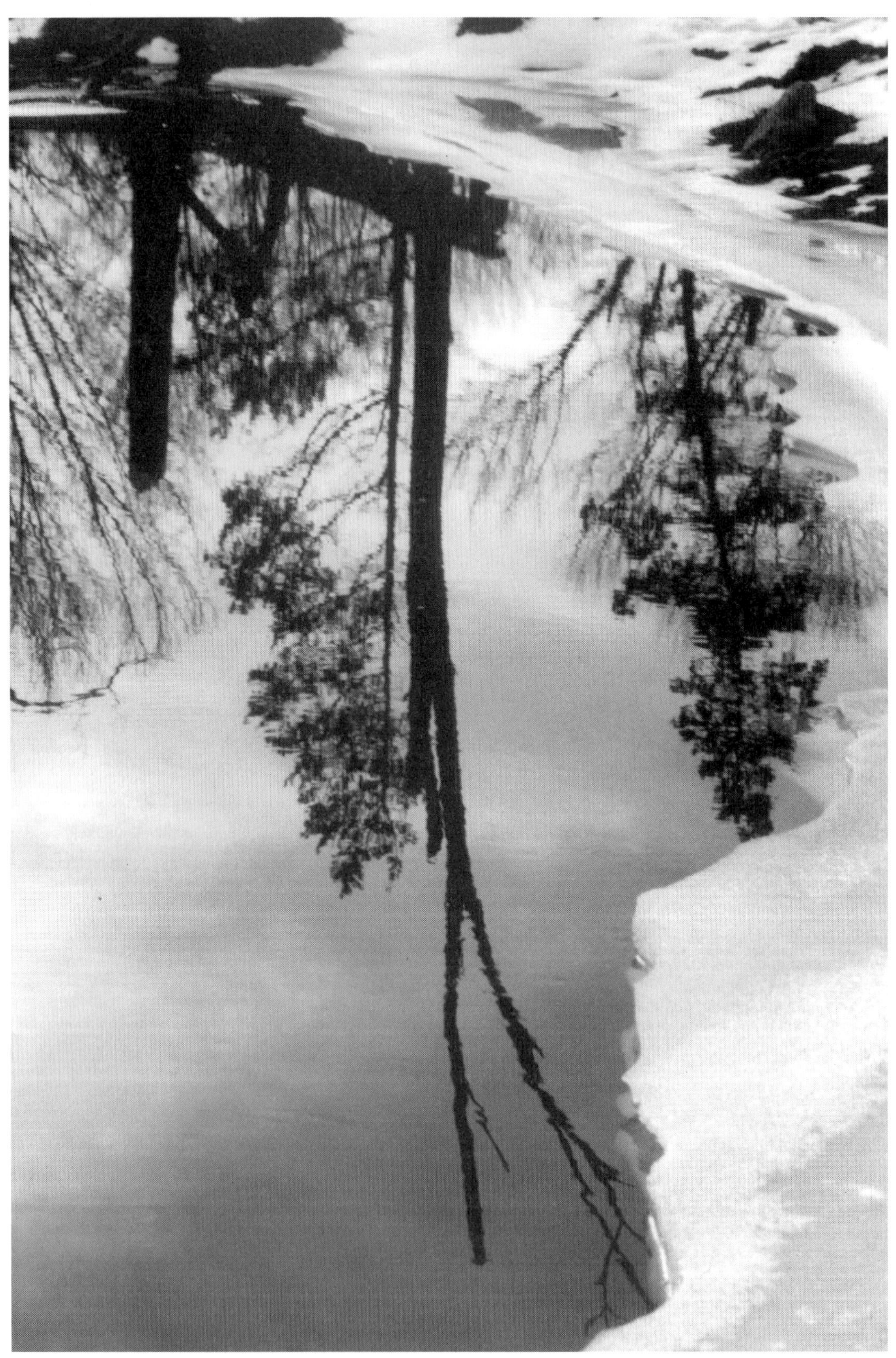

CHAPTER TEN

INHALE, EXHALE

Poses for Difficulties in Breathing

■ ■ ■

BREATHING IS synonymous with life itself. It is the first thing we do at birth and the last thing we do as we die. Yet this natural act is often compromised by conditions that affect breathing, including colds and flu, allergies, asthma, emphysema, postural misalignment, and anxiety.

What is commonly called breathing is technically referred to as respiration. It has three levels. The first is the most familiar: inhaling and exhaling through the nose or mouth. This provides the body with its most precious nutrient, oxygen.

The second level occurs once air has entered the lungs. The lungs contain countless alveolar sacs, which are thin, membranous, microscopic structures shaped like bunches of grapes. In these sacs, two gases—oxygen and carbon dioxide—dance past each other. Oxygen rushes to merge with the oxygen-depleted blood during inhalation, and carbon dioxide and other products of oxidation escape during exhalation.

The third level of respiration occurs at the cellular level, where oxygen is needed for the body's energy production. This process begins when nutrients and oxygen enter each cell and contact certain enzymes. Their interaction liberates the energy necessary for our growth, repair, movement, and thinking.

Respiration is so important to sustaining life that much of the body's energy is devoted to it. If all the alveolar sacs of an adult were spread out flat, they would cover half a tennis court. However, if the skin on the surface of the body of an average adult were spread out flat, it would only cover a space of three yards by three yards. This comparison underscores the prominence the body gives to that exchange of gases we call breathing.

To breathe easily, several conditions must be present. First, the diaphragm, the major muscle of respiration, must move up and down easily with exhalation and inhalation. The intercostal muscles, which connect the ribs, must be free to contract and lift the ribs, as well as relax and let the ribs drop.

Second, some flexibility in the thoracic, or midback, area of the spinal column, is necessary. The thoracic spine moves each time we breathe, back-bending slightly during inhalation and flexing during exhalation.

Below left
FIGURE 10.1
Respiratory System

Below right
FIGURE 10.2
Rib Cage, Front View

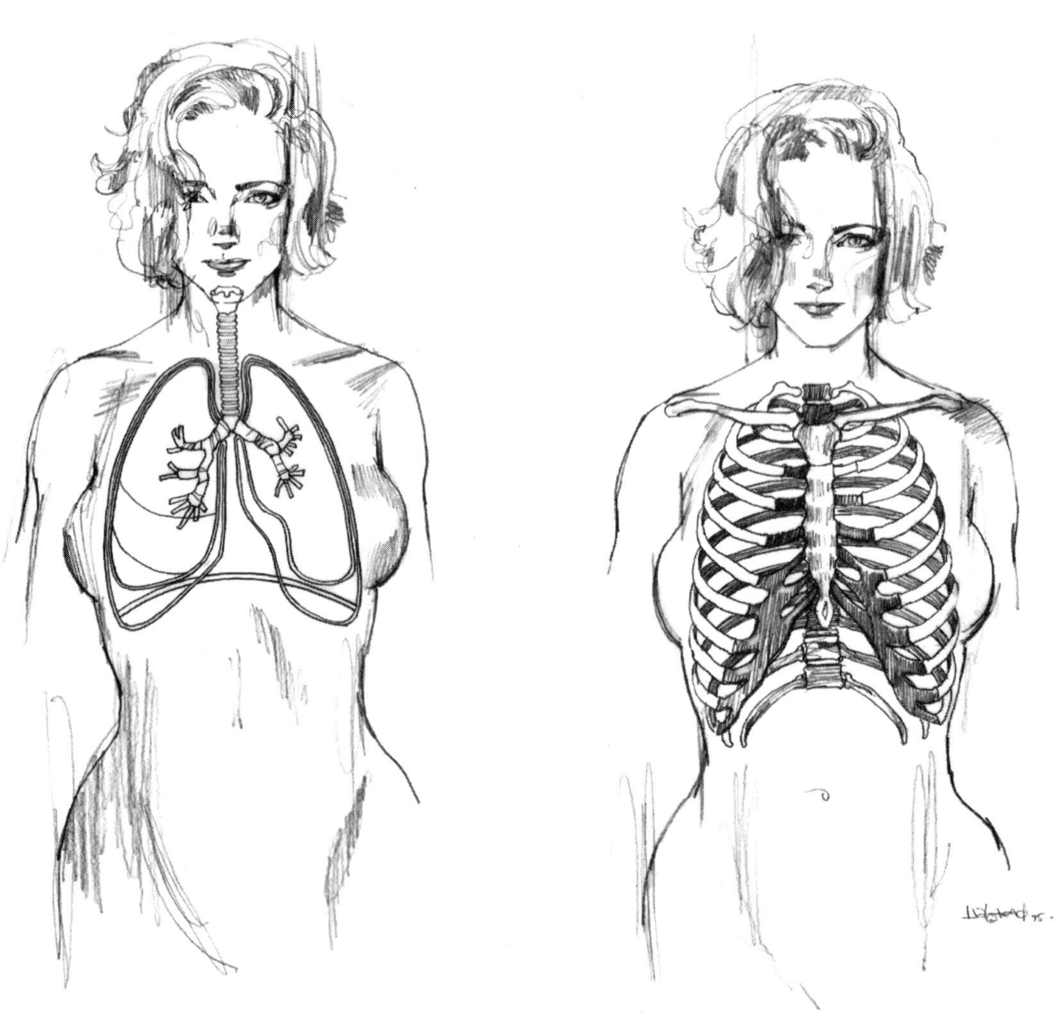

Third, the pectoralis muscles, located at the front top chest, must allow the shoulder girdle to be wide. Tight pectoralis muscles result in the shoulders rolling inward and contribute to the breastbone dropping. This creates a compression of the front chest that limits the movement of the thoracic spine, the intercostals, and the diaphragm, which then limits breathing.

Yoga and the Breath

Modern-day scientists are discovering what yogis have known for thousands of years: yoga movements and breathing techniques increase lung capacity and efficiency, often better than vigorous exercise.[1] Yoga techniques can change the dimensions of the rib cage, thus allowing more air into the lungs. Apparently these movements help to prevent the decrease in flexibility of the rib cage that occurs with age.

Yoga techniques also strengthen the diaphragm muscle. This enables a person to exhale more completely, allowing for a deeper inhalation to follow.

Positively influencing lung capacity not only improves daily life and athletic performance, but it also helps to prevent lung disease due to a decrease in chest mobility. When chest mobility is high, the incidence of respiratory illness is reduced.

The Inhale, Exhale Series

The Inhale, Exhale series is designed to improve your respiratory capacity with gentle stretches to open the chest, create more flexibility in the spine, and relax any emotional tension that restricts your ability to breathe well. It consists of seven poses and takes approximately 45 to 60 minutes. If your time is limited, see the Practice Summary at the end of this chapter for shorter practice sessions using some of the poses from the series.

The Inhale, Exhale series begins with a side-lying pose, to stretch the intercostal muscles and open the ribs, followed by a supported back bend, to open the lungs and stretch the diaphragm and intercostal muscles. Next come two modified inverted poses, to drain the chest of excess fluid, open the lungs, and expand the rib cage. A supported seated pose follows, to lift the diaphragm off the abdominal organs and cool the energy of the lungs. As the series winds down, a supported forward bend comes next. This pose quiets the mind and encourages the lungs and

When one leaf trembles,
the whole bough moves.
—**Chinese Proverb**

diaphragm to move smoothly and freely. As usual, the series concludes with a variation of Basic Relaxation Pose that supports the chest to enhance breathing.

This series is intended for those with mild breathing limitations due to a cold, allergies, asthma, flu, postural misalignment, or anxiety. If you have fever along with your cold or flu, wait until the fever subsides before practicing this series. If you are recovering from pneumonia, surgery on the thoracic cage, or a severe breathing restriction such as emphysema, practice only the Basic Relaxation Pose suggested at the end of the series.

The restorative yoga poses in this chapter are not a substitute for medical treatment. Do not begin this series, any other program in this book, or any other exercise program, until you have had a complete evaluation of your condition by your health care professional. Show this book to your health care professional and discuss the appropriateness of these yoga poses for your condition.

::: PRACTICE

Side-Lying Stretch Pose

Prop

- 2 or more single-fold blankets

Optional Props

- bolster
- clock or timer

Side-Lying Stretch Pose stretches the intercostal muscles on the sides of your body. These muscles help to lift the ribs during normal inhalation and draw the ribs down during strong exhalation. If they are tight, movement of the rib cage is limited, and so is respiration. By stretching the

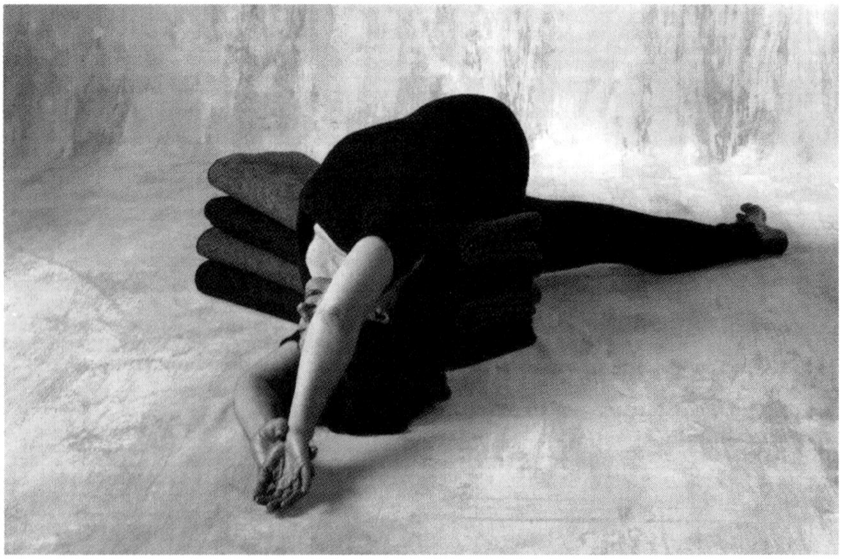

FIGURE 10.3
Side-Lying Stretch Pose

intercostal muscles, breathing is enhanced. This stretching is important if you have had long-term breathing problems, such as asthma.

Setting Up. Lie over a stack of 2 or more single-fold blankets, left side down, so your waist is well-supported at the center of the stack. Neither your hips nor your shoulders should touch the floor. Make sure you are lying exactly on your side, not rolled onto your front or back body.

You grow up the day you have your first real laugh—at yourself.
—Ethel Barrymore

Once in position, you should feel a moderate stretch along the right side of your torso. If you don't, make sure you are lying properly over the stack and are not lying on your shoulder or hip. If you are tall or have a long torso, add 1 or more single-fold blankets on top of the bolster to increase the height before you lie down.

To give an extra stretch to the muscles along the side of your torso and flare open your ribs, raise your arms over your head and let them rest on the floor. Let your head rest on your left arm. To add even more stretch, hold your right wrist with your left hand, gently pulling on your right arm.

Balance the stretch of the arms by stretching the legs. If you practice this stretch, make sure that the distance between the legs is not created by moving one leg or the other but by moving both equally, one to the front and one to the back. Place your top leg, in this case your right leg, on the floor in front of you, so it is 12 to 18 inches from where it was. Move your left leg an equal distance backward. You can enhance this stretch by rolling your right shoulder blade backward to create a diagonally opposed movement to the stretch out through the right leg.

Being There. Take long, slow breaths. Because you are lying on your left side, you will feel your breathing almost exclusively in the right side. Open to the movement of the breath, to the stretch, and to the pleasant feeling that comes from this opening.

In addition to opening the lungs and intercostals on the right, this side-lying pose stimulates the function of the liver. While the liver is not a part of the body you normally associate with stretching and opening, allow it to receive the benefits of Side-Lying Stretch Pose. In addition, allow a healthy stretch to come to the muscles of the hip and side of the thigh.

Coming Back. Practice Side-Lying Stretch Pose on your left side for 30 seconds to 1 minute, gradually increasing the time. When you feel ready, bend your knees and place your right palm on the floor in front of your face. Press the floor and slowly sit up. Turn and lie on your right side to repeat the pose. On this side, you are stimulating the function of the stomach and spleen, located on the left side of your torso.

Once you have practiced for an equal amount of time on the second side, roll onto your back. Keep your pelvis on the bolster and knees bent. In this position, your shoulders will be on the floor. Slide off the bolster in the direction of your head until your lower legs are supported by the bolster (or other props) and your lower back is supported by the floor. Lie here for a few breaths. Roll to one side and slowly sit up.

Benefits. In addition to stretching the intercostal muscles and the diaphragm, this pose stimulates the function of the liver, stomach, and spleen.

Cautions

- If you experience lower back discomfort in this pose, first check your position. Make sure you are lying on your side, with half of your torso on either side of the bolster, rolled neither toward your abdomen nor toward your back. Try the following adjustment: move on the bolster toward your shoulders. If this does not alleviate the discomfort, move the opposite way. If neither relieves the discomfort, skip this pose for now, and go on to the next in the series.

Do not practice this pose:

- if you are more than three months pregnant, during menstruation, or if you have a hiatal hernia.

Mountain Brook Pose

Props

- bolster
- 2 single-fold blankets
- long-roll blanket

Optional Props

- standard-fold blanket
- eyebag
- extra blanket for warmth
- clock or timer

We've all been told to take a deep breath before beginning something challenging. The wisdom here is to center yourself before acting. However, inhaling and exhaling with force can increase anxiety by interfering with efficient oxygen circulation and triggering a panic reaction in the body.[2] To best calm yourself, breathe at your normal rate and volume from the diaphragm. Practice Mountain Brook Pose to open the diaphragm and gain assurance that you can breathe easily.

Setting Up. See page 37 for information on how to set up this pose.

Being There. Breathe normally with eyes closed. Let go of all the parts of your body you use to speak, beginning with the muscles behind your ears, down through the jaw, and all the way to your chin. Allow your

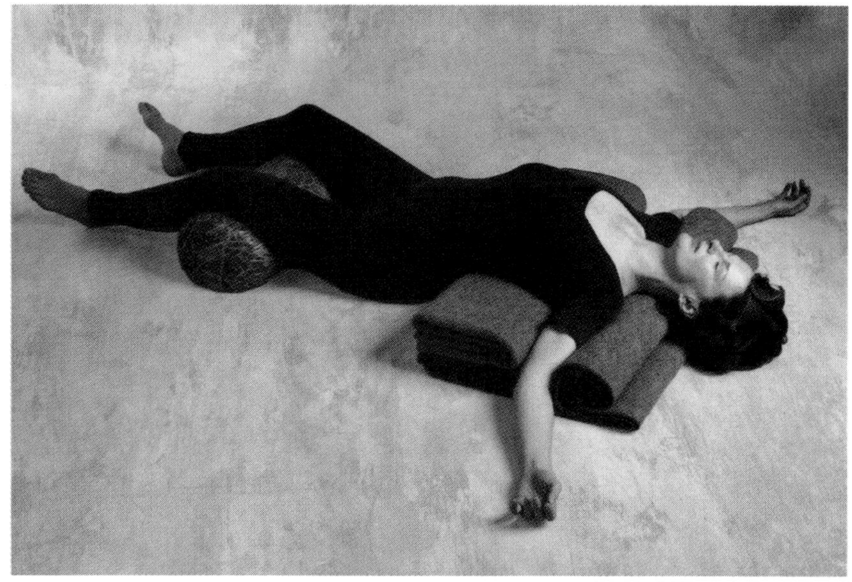

FIGURE 10.4
Mountain Brook Pose

lips to part slightly. Notice any tension in your tongue and throat. Swallow to relax this tension. Give up any unspoken words.

Watch the rise and fall of the breath, noticing if there are any restrictions in the flow. Slowly increase the depth of your inhalation; exhale an equal amount. Breathe up to 10 rounds in this way, so that by the tenth you are breathing deeply and without strain. Now begin to lessen the depth of inhalation and exhalation, taking 10 breaths or fewer to come back to normal breathing. Observe how you feel after the longer breaths and note the difference.

With each exhalation, allow your belly to drop toward your spine. Imagine that your body is softening and spreading. As you continue to relax, you will feel more spacious and loose. Continue to breathe normally, enjoying the freedom you feel in your throat, chest, heart, and belly.

Coming Back. Practice Mountain Brook Pose for 5 minutes. If you are very comfortable or are an experienced yoga student, stay for as long as 15 minutes. If you have a stiff back, start with 1 minute and gradually increase your time in the pose. To come out, remove the eyebag and use your hands to gently lift your head. Then use the support of your hands to slide off the props toward your head. Let your legs rest over the bolster. Lie on the floor for a few minutes before rolling to one side and getting up.

Benefits. Mountain Brook Pose stretches the muscles of respiration, including the diaphragm, intercostals, and abdominals, allowing for easier excursion of the rib cage, especially during inhalation. The back bending movement in the midback opens the front lower ribs, which then allows the lungs to open. In addition, the pose counteracts the slumped sitting posture that so many of our daily activities reinforce, improves digestion, reduces fatigue, and can lift your mood if you feel down.

Caution

- See page 38 for advice on this pose.

Supported Bridge Pose

Props

- 2 bolsters

Optional Props

- 2 or more single-fold blankets
- eyebag
- towel
- extra blanket for warmth
- clock or timer

Supported Bridge Pose exemplifies the essence of restorative yoga. It is relaxing because it is horizontal; it is restorative because it is supported. Use it to enhance your energy and quiet your thoughts.

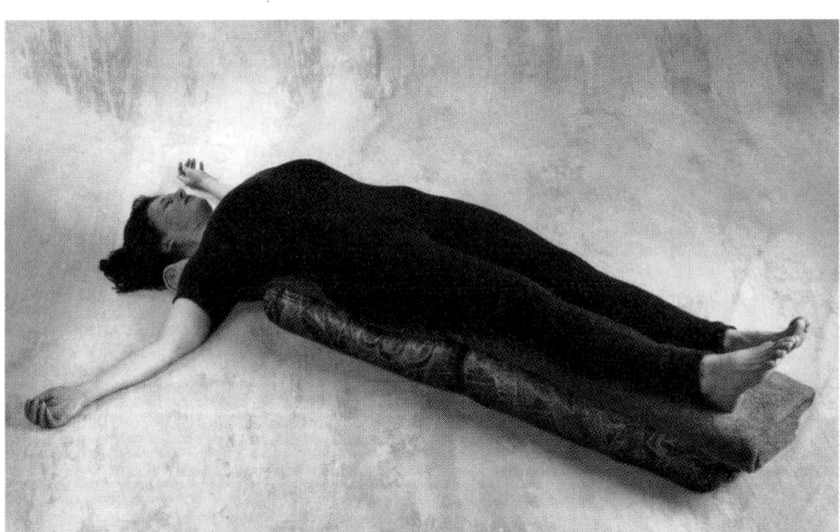

FIGURE 10.5
Supported Bridge Pose

Setting Up. See page 39 for information on how to set up this pose.

Being There. When you have settled comfortably into the props, let your attention rest on your breathing. When you feel ready, begin the Centering Breath (see pages 24 and 26 for complete instructions.) It is important to remember that breathing does not happen only in the middle of the front chest. In this pose, we explore other areas that receive the breath: the rib cage, the upper lungs, and the back.

Begin with the rib cage. As you inhale, feel the lateral movement of your ribs and lungs. Like wings that lift up and out to the sides, the ribs open to make room for the lungs to receive the Centering Breath. Feel the sideways movement as your chest moves toward your arms. As you exhale, feel the ribs and lungs move back to a neutral position. Return to your normal breath for several cycles. Practice the Centering Breath for 2 or 3 rounds, with your attention on the movement of the ribs.

Now bring your awareness to the upper lungs. Feel the freedom of movement that comes as you inhale a Centering Breath. Without straining, welcome more and more breath into the upper lungs, until you feel a pleasant stretch with each breath. Slowly exhale the Centering Breath, and return to several cycles of normal breathing. Stay present with the sensations in the upper lung area for 2 or 3 Centering Breaths. If you feel breathless at any time during this part of practice, return to normal breathing until you feel refreshed, before refocusing on the upper lungs.

For every effect there is a cause.
—**Jamaican Proverb**

As you continue to relax and breathe, move your attention to your back, particularly to your shoulder blades. Inhale a Centering Breath, and notice how this area responds to the breath. Remember, your lungs extend into this area of your back. Allow them to move fully as you exhale a Centering Breath. Return to normal breathing. Stay present to the sensations in your back and around the shoulder blades for 2 or 3 Centering Breaths.

Now simultaneously hold these three areas in your awareness—rib cage, upper lungs, and back—as you receive and release the breath. Practice this for 2 or 3 rounds. Return to normal breathing, and observe the effects of the Centering Breath on your lungs. Enjoy the relaxation that follows.

Coming Back. Practice Supported Bridge Pose for 10 to 12 minutes. To come out, remove the eyebag and slide off the bolsters in the direction of your head. Rest your lower legs on the bolster, with your back on the floor. Stay for a few minutes, then roll to one side. Press down with your hands and sit up slowly.

Benefits. Supported Bridge Pose increases the flexibility of the upper back. It drains fluid from the legs after long periods of standing, thus reducing fatigue. Athletes find it beneficial after a long run to help reduce soreness in the leg and hip muscles. In addition, it is helpful in cases of tension headaches (see chapter 8).

Caution

- See page 40 for advice on this pose.

Elevated Legs-Up-the-Wall Pose

Props

- bolster
- single-fold blanket

Optional Props

- eyebag
- double-fold blanket
- 1 or more single-fold blankets
- standard-fold blanket
- towel
- extra blanket for warmth
- clock or timer

It's commonly known that when you want to relax, you put your feet up. Elevated Legs-Up-the-Wall Pose is a potent example of this proverbial wisdom. Try it. It will help you breathe easier, as it restores your energy and reduces your fatigue.

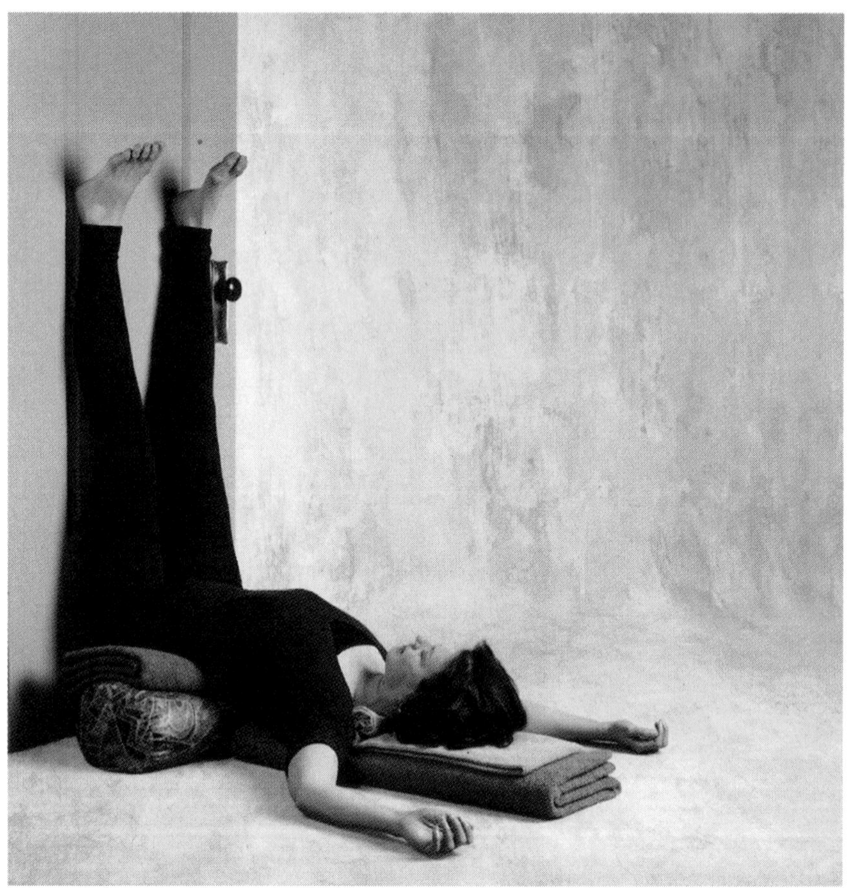

FIGURE 10.6
Elevated Legs-Up-the-Wall Pos

Setting Up. See page 41 for complete instructions on setting up this pose.

Being There. Let yourself be supported by the bolster and the floor. Forget the outside world for a few minutes; allow yourself the important task of doing nothing.

Let each breath be slow and steady, moving it deeply and gently into your lungs and back out. Because your chest is supported in an open position, you may experience a sense of release. Enjoy the sensation of fatigue draining from your legs, your back and shoulders opening, and your mind quieting.

Coming Back. Practice Elevated Legs-Up-the-Wall Pose for up to 10 or 12 minutes. To come out, first remove the eyebag. Then bend your knees, press your feet on the wall, and lift your pelvis slightly. Push the bolster toward the wall with your hands, and slide your body away from the wall by pressing with your feet. Lie on the floor for a few moments, with your lower legs supported by the bolster. Roll to the side and get up slowly.

Benefits. Elevated Legs-Up-the-Wall Pose enhances the ability to breathe by draining the upper respiratory system (in cases of mild congestion), by opening the chest and increasing the flexibility of the upper back, and by stretching the muscles of respiration. It also quiets the mind.

In addition, the pose is particularly useful as an antidote to the systemic effects of stress. It is especially beneficial for those who retain water and whose legs swell easily, and those who have varicose veins or stand for long periods.

Caution

- See page 43 for advice on this inverted pose.

Reclining Hero Pose

When you are unable to breathe well, you might feel an accompanying sense of anxiety, even panic. Reclining Hero Pose can reduce these feel-

Props

- bolster
- 3 single-fold blankets

Optional Props

- 1 to 2 single-fold blankets
- block, book, or blanket
- towel
- eyebag
- extra blanket for warmth
- clock or timer

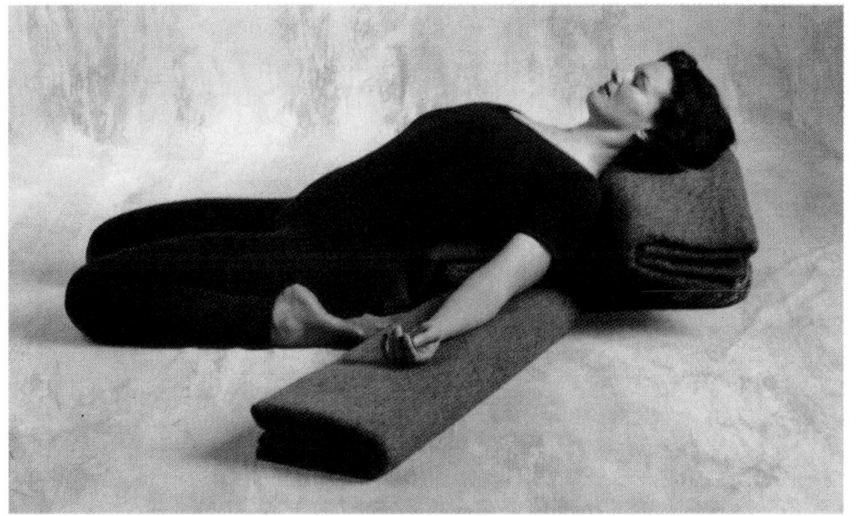

FIGURE 10.7
Reclining Hero Pose

ings by relaxing you and opening the lungs, increasing what is called tidal volume. This is the amount of air you normally inhale and exhale when at rest. When tidal volume is lessened by tightness in the rib cage, asthma, bronchitis, or other causes, there is a buildup of carbon dioxide, or respiratory waste, in the bloodstream. Carbon dioxide acts as an irritant to the nervous system, thus producing anxiety. Use Reclining Hero Pose if you are congested in the upper respiratory area and want to improve your ability to breathe normally while resting.

Setting Up. Before attempting Reclining Hero Pose, determine how comfortable you are in Hero Pose, the seated variation. Kneel with your legs hip-width apart and feet pointing straight back. It is important that your feet are in proper alignment. Sitting in Hero Pose with your feet turned out twists the bones of the lower leg and strains the inner knees.

Gently sit down, with your buttocks resting solidly between your legs on the floor. If you can sit easily and do not feel any discomfort in your knees, ankles, or feet, you can proceed. If not, try the following adjustments. Sit on a block, a book, or a blanket folded into a small bundle. If you feel any discomfort in your knees, come up to a kneeling position. Reach down and gently pull the calf muscles toward your heels, holding them back as you sit down again. This simple movement creates additional space for bending the knees and takes some strain off these joints. If you feel discomfort in your ankles or feet, place a rolled towel under your ankles.

Once you have determined your prop needs, place a single-fold blanket at one end of your bolster, and sit in Hero Pose in front of the other end. Using your hands for support, slowly lie back and rest your torso on the bolster and your head and neck on the single-fold blanket. You can raise the height of the support by adding 1 or more single-fold blankets on top of the bolster. Make sure that your abdomen is comfortable and your chest open. The bottom of your breastbone should lift, not sink. When in position, you should be resting with your torso at a 45-degree angle from the floor. You are not lying flat on your back, but resting halfway between lying and sitting.

The greatest possession
is self-possession.
—Ethel Watts Mumford

Reclining Hero Pose is traditionally practiced with the knees together or nearly together. I recommend that you practice with your knees as close together or as far apart as necessary to make your lower back, knees, and legs comfortable. This may be as little as 6 inches or as much as 14. Spend the time to find the right distance for you.

Cover your eyes with an eyebag. Place each forearm on a single-fold blanket.

Being There. Lying with your hips, legs, and knees in this position may feel unusual at first, so give yourself time to settle in. Let the top of your thighs drop toward the floor.

When your legs feel heavy, your chest will feel lighter and expand more with each breath. With each inhalation, allow the top of your chest to lift and expand horizontally. As you exhale, imagine that the chest does not go back to its position before inhalation but stays lifted and expanded. Each round of breath opens the chest cavity more and more.

If at any time you feel breathless, release all effort to expand the chest, and let your body reestablish its own breathing rhythm. Then slowly begin again to expand the upper chest as you breathe. Each breath can stretch lung tissue, open breathing pathways, and prepare the way for more breaths to come. Remember, the breath is like a visitor, welcomed warmly upon arrival and gently released upon departure.

Every part of an element separated from its mass desires to return to it by the shortest way.
—Leonardo Da Vinci

Coming Back. Practice Reclining Hero Pose for 3 to 4 minutes. As you become accustomed to it, you can practice for up to 10 minutes.

There are two ways to come out of the pose. Option one: Use your arms to lift your torso up and forward, and come onto your hands and knees. Slowly straighten your legs and walk your hands back toward your feet. Bend your knees slightly and stand up slowly. Option two: Use your arms to lift your torso up and forward, and come onto your hands and knees. From this position, put one foot forward. With most of your weight on that foot, stand up as you bring the other foot forward.

Benefits. Reclining Hero Pose opens the upper respiratory tree—the throat, bronchial tubes, and upper lungs. It relieves pressure in the head from sinus problems. In general, Reclining Hero Pose reduces fatigue in the legs from walking and standing. It also relieves indigestion and nausea by lifting the diaphragm off the stomach and liver.

Cautions

- Do not practice Reclining Hero Pose if you feel a sharp pull or pain in or around either knee. If you experience a generalized stretch or a slight ache that resolves itself immediately upon coming out or adjusting your props, it is probably fine to proceed. If difficulty persists, consult your health care professional.
- This pose may cause discomfort in the tops of your feet, especially if you have high arches or tight shin muscles. Try practicing Reclining Hero Pose on your bed.

Supported Crossed-Legs Pose

Prop

- chair

Optional Props

- 1 or more single-fold blankets
- nonskid mat
- extra blanket for warmth
- clock or timer

Because Supported Crossed-Legs Pose places the lungs and muscles of respiration in a relaxed position, this restorative pose is helpful for those with breathing problems. It is a soothing way to associate relaxation with the breathing process.

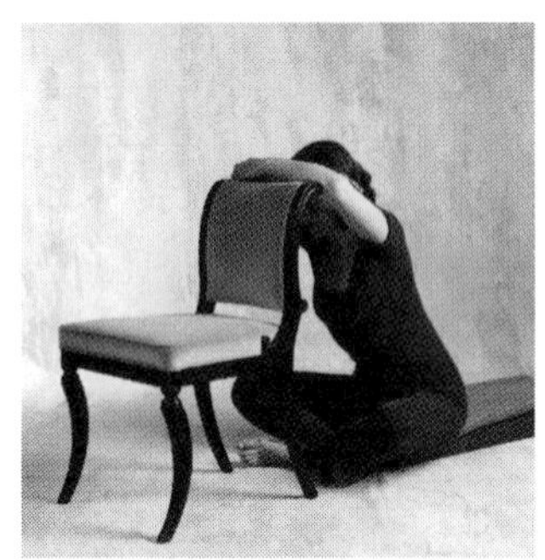

FIGURE 10.9 Supported Crossed-Legs Pose, Variation

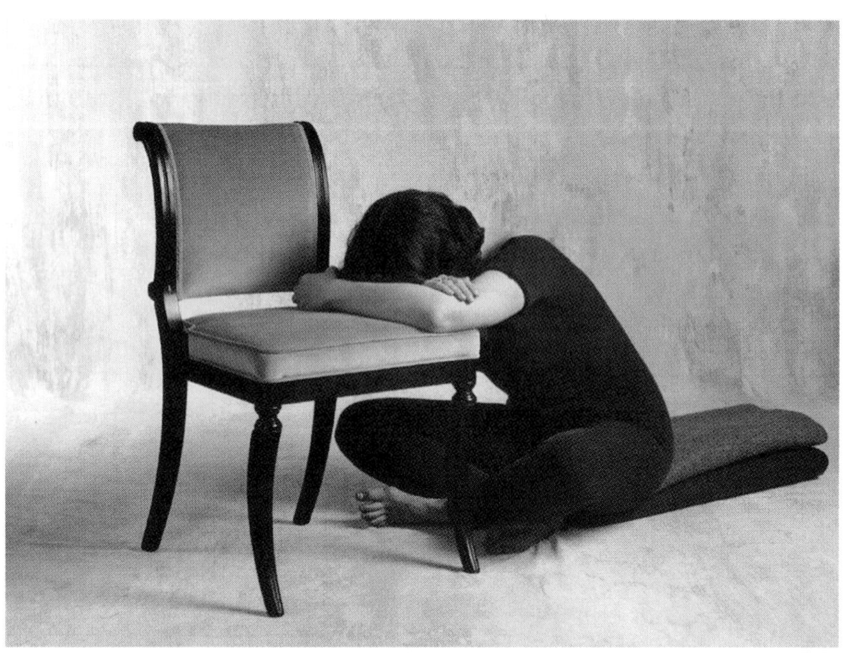

FIGURE 10.8 Supported Crossed-Legs Pose

Setting Up. See page 49 for instructions on how to set up this pose.

Being There. Lean forward and accept the complete support of the chair. Relax your shoulders away from your ears. Imagine that your chest and lungs fall forward, away from the spine.

In this position, we will practice a breathing exercise that focuses on the exhalation. Unless your lungs are empty, they cannot fill with fresh air on the next inhalation. Therefore, to increase your ability to inhale, it is essential to exhale fully.

Begin by taking a slightly longer-than-normal inhalation, and exhale through your nose as slowly as you can. Your exhalation should be longer than your inhalation. Each time you slow the exhalation, you open the respiratory passages in preparation for the next inhalation. If your nose is blocked, exhale through your mouth with your lips pursed like a whistle. After your first long exhalation, take several normal breaths before trying again. Breathe in this way for up to 10 rounds, alternating each extended exhalation with normal breaths. Enjoy the interplay between receiving and surrendering the breath.

Coming Back. Practice Supported Crossed-Legs Pose for 6 to 10 minutes. Remember to practice for an equal amount of time with each ankle crossed on top of the other. If you are practicing with your head turned to the side, turn it to the opposite side for an equal amount of time.

To come out, slowly sit up and lean back on your hands to relieve any strain on your back. If you feel any discomfort in your back, lie on the floor with your calves resting on the chair for a few minutes. (If you are more than three months pregnant, lie on your side.)

Benefits. Supported Crossed-Legs Pose frees the lungs and opens the front body so that the diaphragm is not restricted. The breathing exercise of slowed exhalation forces open the small passageways of the lungs, allowing a more complete inhalation. Those having a mild asthma attack may benefit from practicing this pose during the attack. It not only helps to increase the amount of air going into and out of the lungs, but it also helps to reduce the anxiety produced by not being able to breathe well.

Cautions

- At no time during breathing practice should you feel breathless, not even slightly. If you do, return to normal breathing until any hunger for air is satiated or agitation is resolved. When you feel ready, begin the long inhalation again, with the slow exhalation through your nose or pursed lips.
- See page 50 for more advice on this pose.

Basic Relaxation Pose with Chest Elevated

The Inhale, Exhale series concludes with a variation of Basic Relaxation Pose, in which your body is supported by three blankets. The first blanket supports your back and chest, the second supports your head, and the third supports your legs. You may find it easier to breathe in this position because your chest is higher than the abdomen. In addition, this variation of Basic Relaxation Pose reduces the tendency to cough that lying flat on your back makes worse.

Props

- 2 single-fold blankets
- long-roll blanket

Optional Props

- eyebag
- extra blanket for warmth
- clock or timer

Setting Up. Sit in front of the short end of a single-fold blanket, with it touching your hips. Place another single-fold blanket at the other end

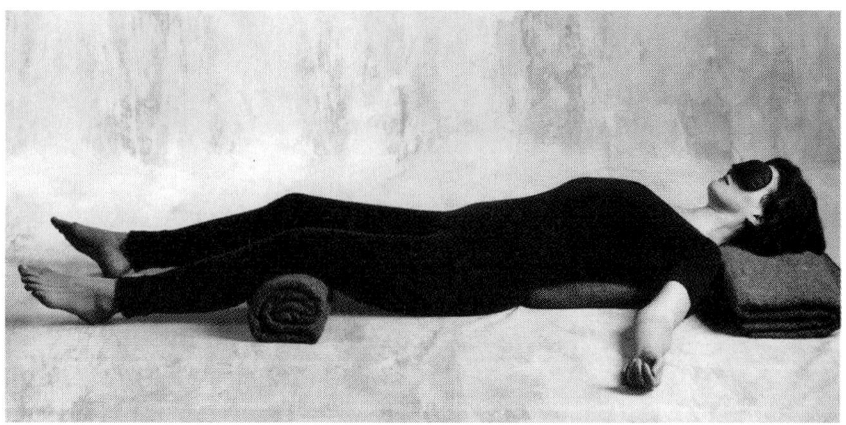

FIGURE 10.10
Basic Relaxation Pose
with Chest Elevated

to support your head. Position a long-roll blanket to support your knees. If you need an extra blanket for warmth, cover yourself. Lie back over the props. You head should be higher than your chest, and your chest higher than your abdomen. Place the eyebag on your eyes.

Once you have established yourself, take a moment to observe the position of your body. Your arms and legs should be equidistant from an imaginary line drawn from the tip of your nose down to exactly midway between the feet. Most people practice with the palms turned up, but if this is not comfortable, turn them down and let the elbows relax. The most important thing is that you feel completely at ease and supported by the props and the floor.

Being There. See page 26 for guidance on being in the pose. Whatever your breathing difficulty, imagine that for at least the next several minutes, your breath is smooth and silky. The inhalation flows in and the exhalation melts away. There is no resistance to this natural rhythm. Focus on the pleasing quality of the breath, and let the volume take care of itself.

Coming Back. Practice Basic Relaxation Pose with Chest Elevated for 10 to 15 minutes. Slowly bend one knee, then the other, and gently roll onto your side. Let the eyebag fall off by itself. Open your eyes when you are ready. Rest in this position for a few breaths. To sit up, press the floor with the elbow of your lower arm and the palm of the upper hand. Take a few breaths before standing up and resuming your normal activities.

Benefits. This variation of Basic Relaxation Pose reduces the fatigue and anxiety that often accompany breathing difficulties.

Caution

- If you are more than three months pregnant, practice Side-Lying Relaxation Pose in chapter 13.

PRACTICE SUMMARY

45 to 60 Minutes

POSE	TIME
Side-Lying Stretch Pose	1 to 2 minutes
Mountain Brook Pose	5 minutes
Supported Bridge Pose	10 to 12 minutes
Elevated Legs-Up-the-Wall Pose	10 to 12 minutes
Reclining Hero Pose	3 to 4 minutes
Supported Crossed-Legs Pose	6 to 10 minutes
Basic Relaxation Pose with Chest Elevated	10 to 15 minutes

20 Minutes

POSE	TIME
Supported Bridge Pose	5 minutes
Supported Crossed-Legs Pose	5 minutes
Basic Relaxation Pose with Chest Elevated	10 minutes

30 Minutes

POSE	TIME
Mountain Brook Pose	5 minutes
Elevated Legs-Up-the-Wall Pose	10 minutes
Basic Relaxation Pose with Chest Elevated	15 minutes

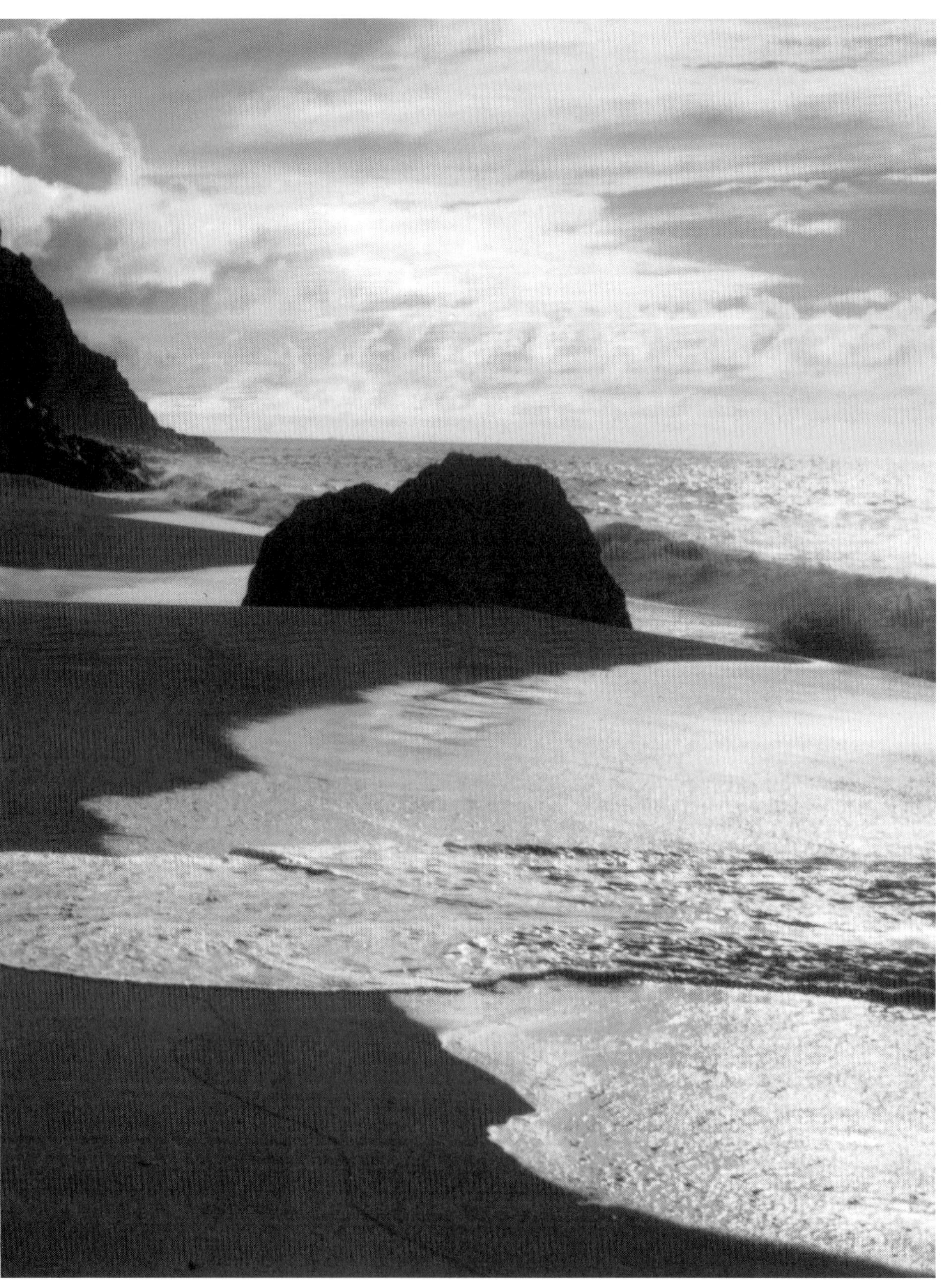

CHAPTER ELEVEN

DISTURBED RHYTHMS

Poses for Jet Lag

TRAVELING LONG DISTANCES in a relatively short period of time is at the root of the constellation of symptoms commonly called jet lag. According to doctors who have studied jet lag, the most common symptoms are drowsiness, a tendency to fall asleep during the day, or conversely, the inability to fall asleep at night or a tendency to wake up too early in the morning. Not only are these symptoms unpleasant and inconvenient, but they may be accompained by a lessened ability to think clearly and concentrate, as well as disturbances in digestion and elimination.[1]

The body aches that accompany jet lag result from sitting upright in a confined space for many hours and breathing recycled air. Your feet may swell, your lower back may ache, and you may experience sinus problems from dry air and the change in air pressure.

Technically jet lag is caused by travel across several time zones, so that your circadian, or twenty-four-hour, biological rhythm that controls your body is not in harmony with the time at your destination. Therefore, jet lag occurs when you travel from east to west or vice versa; it does not occur when you travel north-south without crossing time zones. If you feel symptoms from this direction of travel, it is probably due mainly to fatigue and poor air quality.

How long it takes to recover from jet lag is individual and depends on several factors. First, recovery is relative to how many time zones you crossed. Obviously, it takes longer to get back to normal if you have traveled over eight time zones.

Second, direction of travel is another variable. For most people, traveling east is more difficult because a normal 7 A.M. wake-up time in the new time zone will actually be 2 A.M. body time if you have crossed five time zones. When you travel west, getting up at 7 A.M. is like sleeping in until noon as far as your body is concerned.

The final factor influencing recovery from jet lag is tied to individual physiology. Simply put, some people adapt more quickly to the new time.

Take Care in the Air

> To change your mind is to change your body, to function differently.
> —STANLEY KELEMAN

In addition to restorative yoga, here are some simple strategies you can implement during air travel to reduce the effects of jet lag.

- Eat less than normal. After all, you are not burning off many calories by sitting.
- Avoid alcoholic beverages, but do drink a glass of liquid, preferably water, for every hour you are on the plane.
- Walk up and down the aisle to get some exercise. This will decrease stiffness and increase circulation.
- Bring an inflatable neck pillow and eye mask. Even if you don't sleep, the added comfort will help you rest. If you don't have these travel items, ask the flight attendant for a blanket. Roll the blanket to a comfortable thickness, and place between your neck and the seat back.
- Do some simple stretches at the back of the plane while you are waiting for your turn in the bathroom. For example, try Half Wall Hang from chapter 13. Even if you are not pregnant, this is a great stretch, especially when space is limited.
- Apply the suggestions for sitting well described in chapter 17.

The Disturbed Rhythms Series

The Disturbed Rhythms series will relieve the effects of jet lag and help you have a more pleasant travel experience. It consists of seven poses and takes approximately 40 to 55 minutes. It begins with an inversion to reduce swelling in the legs from prolonged sitting, followed by a back bend to alleviate back discomfort. This back bend will also prepare you for the two inversions that follow. These inversions are to calm and refresh your mind. A reclining pose comes next to relax you deeply.

A supported forward bend follows. This pose stretches the back and inner thighs, which often tighten during prolonged sitting. The Disturbed Rhythms series concludes with Basic Relaxation Pose. In this variation, the legs are elevated to relieve swelling and reduce general fatigue.

Guidelines for practicing the Disturbed Rhythms series are simple. Once you have arrived at your destination, I recommend three things:

- Assume the schedule of the new time zone right away. Set your watch and alarm clock to the new time, and try to rise, eat, work, and sleep in step with your new home base.
- Expose yourself to at least 30 minutes of early morning light as soon as possible after arrival. This will help to reset your biological rhythms.
- Practice the Disturbed Rhythms series as soon as possible after arrival, and again first thing the next morning. In addition, set aside some practice time each day during your trip, perhaps in the late afternoon or early evening. You will find that this series not only relieves jet lag, but it also helps with fatigue from a day of sightseeing or business meetings.

If your time or access to props is limited, see the Practice Summary at the end of the chapter for suggestions. This series can also be used for the first few days after you return home.

Have Mat, Will Travel

The poses in the Disturbed Rhythms series are described using the props common to the rest of the book. If you have an eyebag, an elastic bandage, and the nonskid variety of yoga mat, bring them along (see Resources). The mat folds, and the eyebag and elastic bandage are small; all will tuck easily into your suitcase. The mat can substitute for a blanket or head support, and it's a clean and portable surface for practicing.

Art, it seems to me, should simplify.
—Willa Cather

I realize that few of us travel with a bolster or blankets. Look around your hotel room and be creative. Use whatever is convenient to help you take care of yourself. Here are some suggestions:

- Use the bedspread as a bolster or blanket alternative.
- Use bath towels to support your head and neck. For example, substitute a hotel bath towel for the standard-fold blanket. Fold it lengthwise, then in half, then in half again. Roll slightly and place in the curve of your neck.

- Try the telephone directory or other books to fill in as props.
- Use detachable chair cushions.
- Request an extra blanket or two from the front desk.
- Do the poses on the bed if the floor does not seem clean enough to lie on.

::: PRACTICE

Legs-Up-the-Wall Pose

Prop
- wall

Optional Props
- standard-fold blanket
- eyebag
- clock or timer

If you removed your shoes during the flight, you may have noticed that it is harder to get them back on because your feet have swollen. Swelling is caused by sitting for long periods with your legs hanging down. Practice Legs-Up-the-Wall Pose as soon as possible after arriving at your destination to relieve your discomfort. If you have time for

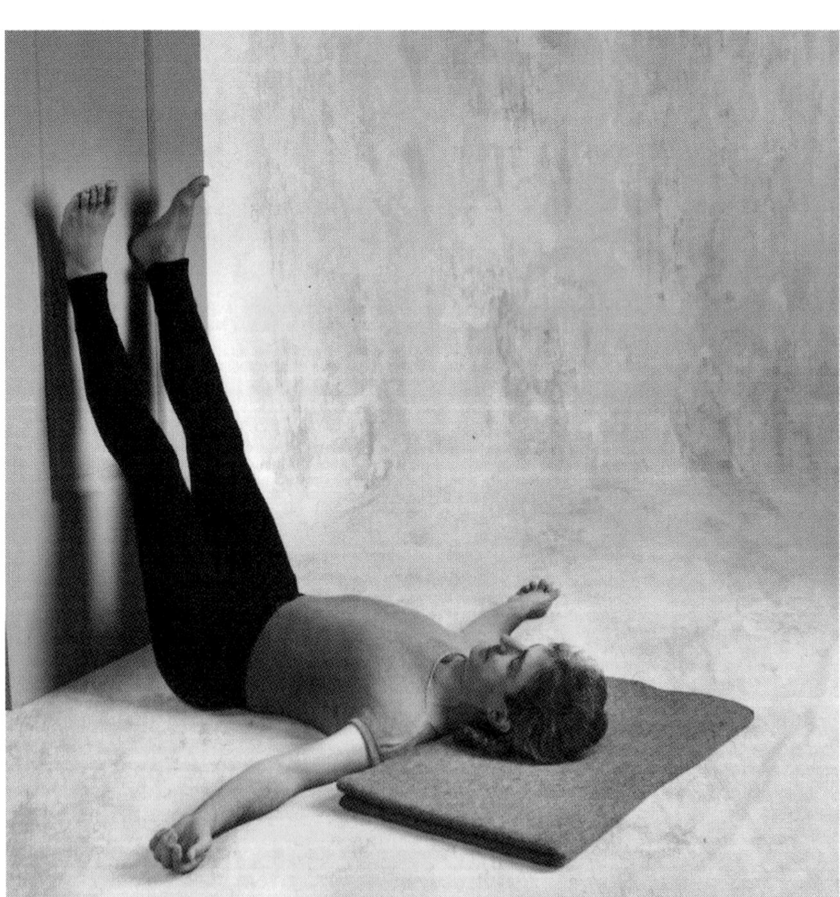

FIGURE 11.1
Legs-Up-the-Wall Pose

only one pose from this series, do this one daily. In fact, do it several times a day.

Setting Up. See page 56 for instructions on setting up this pose.

Being There. After hours of sitting upright with your legs hanging down, few positions feel as good as this one. Take several long, slow breaths. As you do, imagine the accumulated fluid in your legs flowing down toward the abdomen. With it, all tension drains out of your legs. They begin to feel lighter and softer. Imagine that your brain is shrinking in size as it moves away from your forehead and sinks toward the back of your head and the floor. Feel your entire spine supported by the floor. The position of the arms creates a feeling of being open and free. Welcome the opportunity to be still.

Adventure is worthwhile in itself.
—Amelia Earhart

Coming Back. Practice Legs-Up-the-Wall Pose for 4 to 7 minutes, longer if you are comfortable. When ready, remove the eyebag and open your eyes. Rest for a few breaths before bending your knees toward your chest and rolling to one side. Pause again for a few breaths before slowly coming to a sitting position with the help of your arms.

Benefits. Legs-Up-the-Wall Pose reduces swelling and fatigue in the legs. Practice it to help recover from jet lag, as well as from fatigue from walking, standing, and sitting while sightseeing.

Cautions

- If you experience strain at the back of your knees in this pose, try these variations. Move closer to the wall, so that your legs are more perpendicular. If you are already close to the wall and the strain persists, bend your knees several inches. If this does not alleviate the strain, move about 12 inches away from the wall and bend your knees, resting the soles of your feet on the wall.
- See page 57 for more advice on this inverted pose.

Simple Supported Back Bend

Props

- bolster
- long-roll blanket

Optional Props

- eyebag
- block
- double-fold blanket
- extra blanket for warmth
- clock or timer

Airline seats seats, like most chairs, are designed to accommodate the average body, someone who is five feet six in height. Few of us fall into that category, either because we are taller or shorter or because our torso and leg-length ratio makes sitting in these seats uncomfortable. When I walk up and down the aisle of the airplane, the only "average" I notice is that most passengers sit with the front of the body collapsed and head thrust forward. Simple Supported Back Bend counteracts this collapsed sitting position by lengthening and opening the chest and throat. It also prepares the body for the inversions that follow.

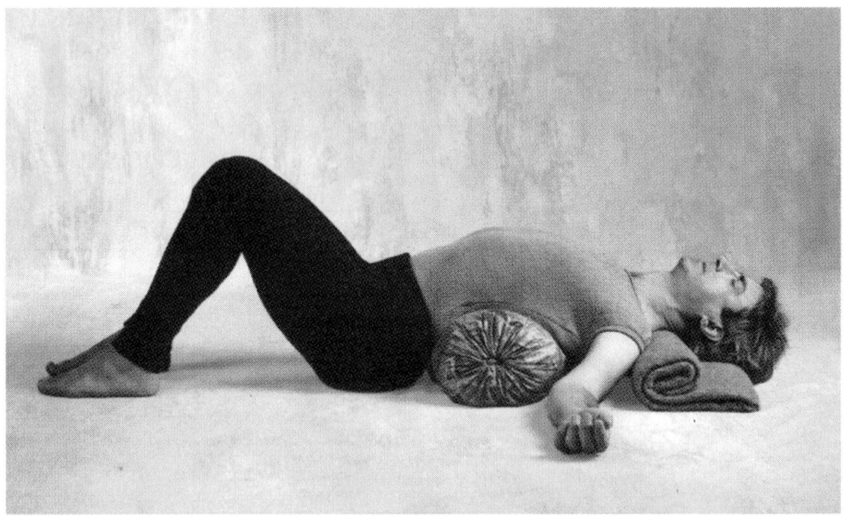

FIGURE 11.2
Simple Supported Back Bend

Setting Up. See page 31 for instructions on how to set up this pose.

Being There. When you set down a heavy suitcase, you feel release in your tired arm muscles and relief at having finally arrived at your destination. Imagine that your entire body is this heavy suitcase; lay it down and let it open to the relaxing benefits of Simple Supported Back Bend.

Breathe slowly and evenly. Feel held by the props. Your arms are wide open and free. With each inhalation, your front body opens; with each exhalation, your belly and organs soften, your back muscles release, and your mind quiets. As you continue to relax, allow your back to sink into the props and your chest to open slowly, as your spine adapts to this new position.

Coming Back. Practice Simple Supported Back Bend for 2 to 3 minutes. To come out, remove the eyebag. Push with your feet and slide off the bolster toward your head. Rest for a few breaths, with your lower back flat on the floor and your legs supported by the bolster. Roll to the side and sit up slowly.

Benefits. Simple Supported Back Bend will leave you feeling refreshed. It improves breathing, reduces fatigue, and counters the negative effects of long travel on the spine, especially the midback area.

Caution

- See page 33 for more advice on this back bend.

Elevated Legs-Up-the-Wall Pose

I remember as a child how I would sometimes lie on my back and hang my upper body off my parents' bed, watching an upside-down world from this comfortable position. Little did I realize that I was actually

Props

- bolster
- single-fold blanket

Optional Props

- elastic bandage or alternative
- double-fold blanket
- 1 or more single-fold blankets
- standard-fold blanket
- towel
- extra blanket for warmth
- clock or timer

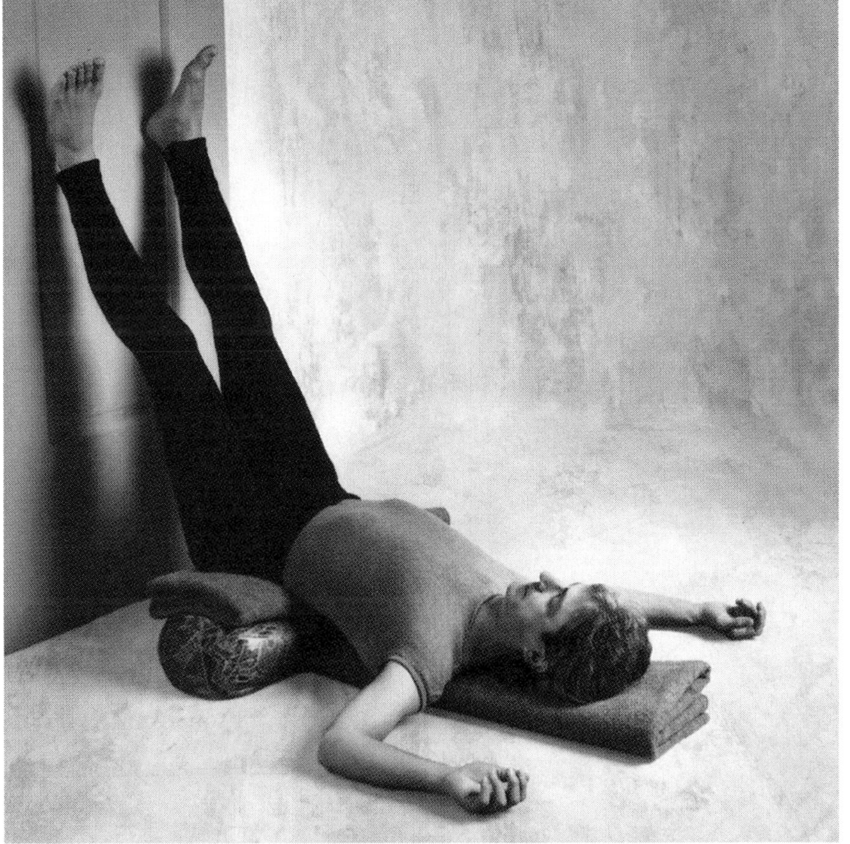

FIGURE 11.3
Elevated Legs-Up-the-Wall Pose

practicing a restorative yoga pose—one that opened my chest with a back bend and elevated my legs and pelvis.

While putting your legs up certainly reduces swelling and tiredness in your legs, elevating the abdomen and opening the chest adds the benefits of an inversion and a back bend to a travel-weary body. In this variation, I recommend wrapping your head with an elastic bandage.

Setting Up. See page 41 for a full discussion of setting up this pose; see page 89 for instructions on how to use the head wrap and alternatives. If you use a head wrap, be sure you can smoothly roll back and swing your legs up the wall. Put on the head wrap before doing so. If you prefer an alternative to the elastic bandage, put it in position once you are in the pose.

Being There. Breathe slowly, steadily, and easily. Allow yourself to receive the support of the wall, the bolster, and the floor. Embrace the feelings of release, as your back and shoulders open. Enjoy the sensations in your legs, as fatigue drains away. Relax as your mind quiets.

Coming Back. Practice Elevated Legs-Up-the-Wall Pose for 5 to 9 minutes, or longer if you are comfortable. If you are using an alternative to the head wrap, remove it now. Lie still for several breaths before opening your eyes.

Bend your knees, press your feet on the wall, and lift your pelvis up a little. Push the bolster toward the wall with your hands, and slide your body away from the wall by pressing with your feet. Lie on the floor a few moments, with your lower legs supported by the bolster. Then roll to the side and get up slowly. If you are using a head wrap, remove it now. Sit quietly for several breaths before opening your eyes.

Humor brings insight and tolerance.
—Agnes Repplier

Benefits. Elevated Legs-Up-the-Wall Pose relieves the systemic effects of stress, particularly those caused by long hours of sitting on an airplane. It opens the chest and refreshes the heart and lungs. With the head wrapped, it quiets the mind and allows you to drop into a more deeply relaxed state. In addition, this pose is especially beneficial for those who retain water and whose legs swell easily, and those who have varicose veins or stand for long periods.

Caution

- See page 43 for more advice on this pose.

Supported Bridge Pose

With jet lag, your body and mind feel as though they're still back home. Let this restorative pose bridge the gap between past and present, and connect you to your new place and rhythm.

Props
- 2 bolsters

Optional Props
- 2 or more single-fold blankets
- eyebag
- towel
- extra blanket for warmth
- clock or timer

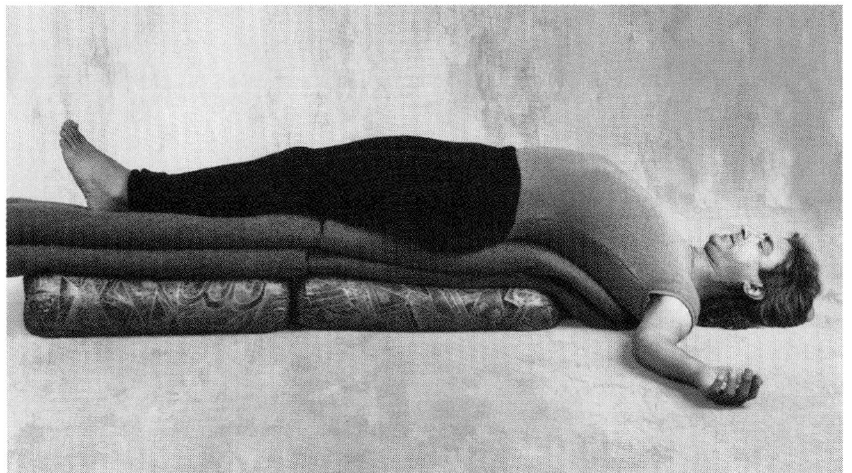

FIGURE 11.4
Supported Bridge Pose

Setting Up. See page 39 for a complete description of how to set up this pose.

Being There. Begin by making sure that you are comfortable. Enjoy the feeling that you can finally stretch out, no longer confined by the small space of an airline seat. Gently bring your attention to your breathing. Feel the lateral movement of your lungs and ribs with each inhalation and exhalation. As you continue to breathe, let your upper back curl around the bolster, opening gradually to the back bend. Release all the tension that accumulated from sitting for so long.

To enhance your relaxation, let your eyeballs turn downward. Let the energy of thought draw inward, as the energy of the body opens and expands.

Coming Back. Practice Supported Bridge Pose for 8 minutes or more, as long as you are comfortable. To come out, remove the eyebag and slide off the bolsters in the direction of your head. Rest your lower legs on the bolster with your back on the floor. Stay for a few minutes, and then roll to one side. Press down with your hands, and sit up slowly.

Benefits. A modified inversion, Supported Bridge Pose drains fluid from the legs, thus reducing fatigue. It quiets the mind and relieves the discomfort of sitting with the shoulders rounded forward. In addition, this pose is helpful in cases of headache (see chapter 8) or mental agitation, which are often the symptoms of overwork.

Caution

- See page 40 for advice on this inverted pose.

Supported Bound-Angle Pose

Props

- bolster
- 4 long-roll blankets
- double-fold blanket
- belt or sandbag

Optional Props

- single-fold blanket
- eyebag
- extra blanket for warmth
- clock or timer

Travel tip: If you are without a belt or sandbag, practice this pose near a wall or chest of drawers. Position yourself so that your feet touch the wall and they will not slide.

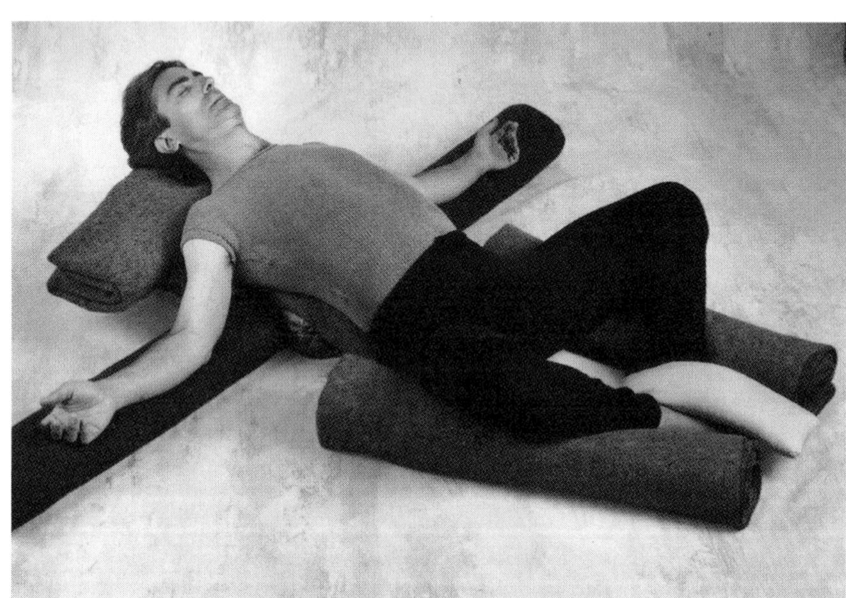

FIGURE 11.5
Supported Bound-Angle Pose

Setting Up. See page 34 for complete instructions on setting up this pose.

Being There. Travel is fatiguing, whether or not you have jet lag. As you settle into the props, allow yourself to feel the fatigue completely. It may feel worse at first, but as you relax, the fatigue will begin to lift.

When you feel this lift, begin the Centering Breath. (See pages 24 and 26 for practice instructions.)

Coming Back. Practice Supported Bound-Angle Pose for 8 to 9 minutes, or longer if you are comfortable. Some individuals prefer to make this pose the focus of their restorative practice and remain as long as 30 minutes. After relaxing so deeply, let the outside world come slowly into your awareness. Take in the sounds around you; pay attention to the sensations of your body.

As you feel ready, remove the eyebag and slowly open your eyes. To come up, press down with your arms, and sit up slowly. Undo the belt or remove the sandbag from your feet. Slowly stretch the legs out in front of you to release any tension in the knees. Carefully move to the next pose or on to the rest of your day.

Benefits. Supported Bound-Angle Pose gently stretches the legs and relaxes the abdomen, which is decidedly beneficial after having been confined to an airline seat. The pose also relaxes the intestines, helping the traveler avoid constipation. Because you practice it on the floor, Supported Bound-Angle Pose can help you feel grounded in the here and now.

In general, those who have high blood pressure and breathing problems often find this pose especially pleasant. It is also beneficial for women during the menstrual period (see chapter 12) and during menopause (see chapter 14).

Caution

- See pages 35 and 36 for advice on this pose.

Supported Seated-Angle Pose

Prop

- bolster

Optional Props

- chair
- 1 or more single-fold blankets
- towel
- extra blanket for warmth
- clock or timer

Perhaps train travel—with sleeping compartments, the rhythm of the rails, and crossing time zones slowly—was a more healthful way to travel. But the demands of business travel and limited vacation time have largely replaced the train with the airplane. My fantasy is to travel on an airplane where I have a bed and can sleep during the flight, arriving at my destination completely rested. Since this is unlikely, I practice Supported Seated-Angle Pose as part of my restorative sequence shortly after arriving to support myself with privacy and rest.

Setting Up. See page 46 for complete instructions on setting up this pose.

Being There. Breathe normally. Let your body be completely supported by the props. Let your abdomen and chest soften, as you breathe easily

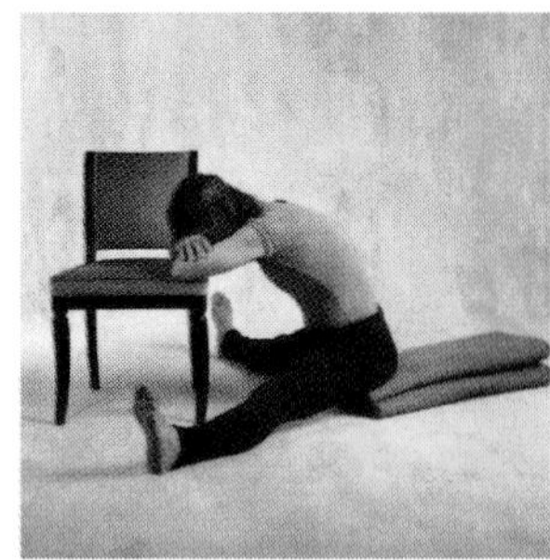

FIGURE 11.7
Supported Seated-Angle Pose, Variation

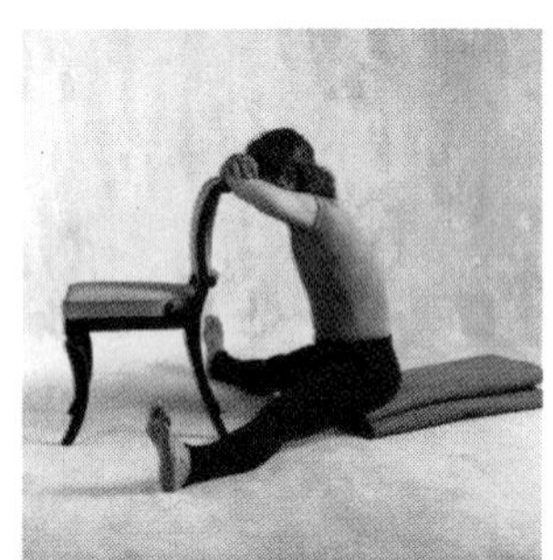

FIGURE 11.8
Supported Seated-Angle Pose, Variation

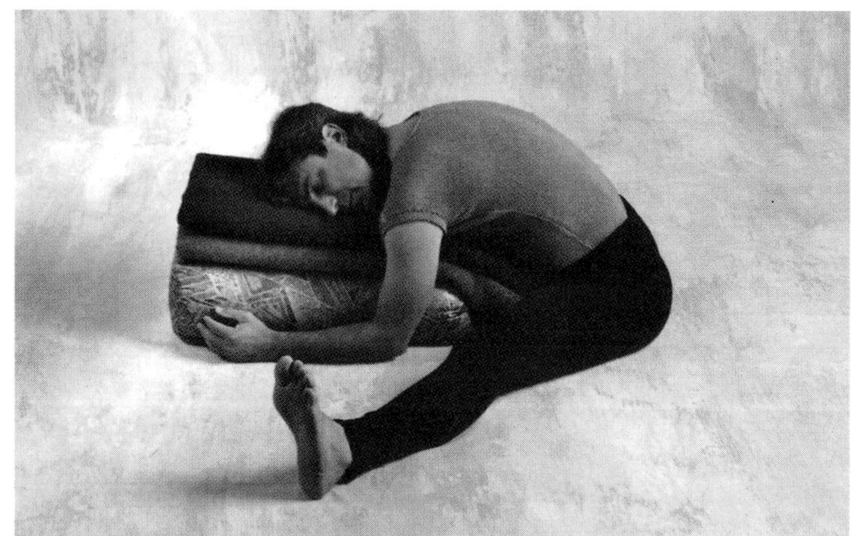

FIGURE 11.6 Supported Seated-Angle Pose

and freely. Feel only the sensations of your body, as the external world fades away. Let your travel fatigue melt away. There is no longer any need to cope with the tasks required to get you here. Enjoy yourself, letting the pose restore you.

Coming Back. Practice Supported Seated-Angle Pose for 3 to 4 minutes. Come up slowly and lean back on your arms for several breaths to relieve your back.

Benefits. A forward bend, Supported Seated-Angle Pose soothes the nervous system and quiets the mind. It can be practiced to relieve tension headaches (see chapter 8) or insomnia (see chapter 9). The pressure on the forehead enhances relaxation, especially important if you are fatigued from travel.

In general, forward bends quiet the organs of digestion and elimination, such as the stomach, intestines, and liver, which are located in the front of the body. They balance the squeezing effect that back bends have on the spine and kidneys and open the lower back area. This is important, especially if your lower back feels tight from sitting for long hours strapped in an airline seat.

Women often find this pose helpful during menstruation and throughout pregnancy. If you are pregnant, make sure there is room between the chair and your belly, so that you and the baby are comfortable.

Caution

- See page 48 for advice on this pose.

Basic Relaxation Pose with Legs Elevated

Basic Relaxation Pose can help you experience what your body has been craving for hours: relaxation. This pose places the least metabolic demand possible on your body, except for when you sleep. By practicing it, not only do you eliminate your travel fatigue, but you also relax so you can sleep when you need to.

Props

- standard-fold blanket
- 3 or more single-fold blankets

Optional Props

- sandbag
- eyebag
- extra blanket for warmth
- clock or timer

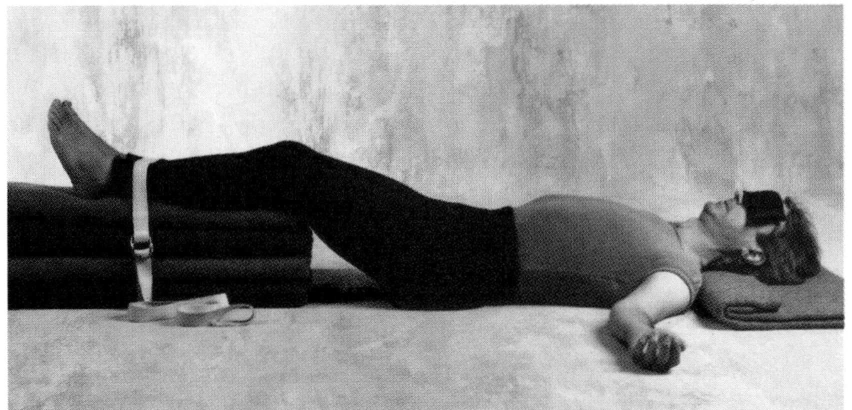

FIGURE 11.9
Basic Relaxation Pose with Legs Elevated

Setting Up. See page 25 for a complete description of setting up Basic Relaxation Pose. As in the basic pose, before you lie down, position a standard-fold blanket for your head and neck to rest on. In this variation, you also stack 2 or more single-fold blankets to elevate your lower legs at least 10 to 12 inches and to support their length.

Begin by sitting on the floor and placing your lower legs on the stack of single-fold blankets. You can place a sandbag across your ankles to anchor your legs on the blankets. (Alternatively, use a strap to secure your legs. Place it under the blankets and over your legs, just below the knees.) If you have a tendency to get cold, cover your legs with an unfolded blanket. Use the strength and support of your arms to help you lie back.

Roll the long edge of your standard-fold blanket slightly, to support the gentle curve of your neck. Adjust the prop placement under your head and neck, so you are comfortable. Your chin should be slightly lower than your forehead. This position quiets the frontal lobes of the brain. If you are using an extra blanket for warmth, pull it up to cover your torso and arms. Cover your eyes with an eyebag. Rest your arms by the sides of your body.

Being There. You have arrived. All the preparations for travel are over, and the effort to get to your destination is past. Allow yourself to enjoy finally being here. There is nowhere to go now. Let the floor support you completely, as you unwind.

When you feel ready, begin the Centering Breath. Refer to pages 24 and 26 for guidance in this breathing awareness technique. Practice the Centering Breath for 10 rounds. When you are finished, rest in the here and now. Savor the silence.

Coming Back. Practice Basic Relaxation Pose with Legs Elevated for 10 to 15 minutes. To come out of the pose, move as slowly as necessary to maintain your relaxation. Exhale as you bend one knee, then the other, and bring them toward your chest. Roll to one side. Rest in this position for a few breaths. To sit up, press the floor with the elbow of your lower arm and the palm of the upper hand. Sit quietly for a few breaths before standing up and resuming your normal activities.

Benefits. This variation of Basic Relaxation Pose reduces fatigue, reduces swelling in the legs and feet, soothes the nerves, and eases mental agitation. It relieves many of the little aches and pains that come with living in a body, which are made worse by jet travel.

Caution

- If you are more than three months pregnant, practice Side-Lying Relaxation Pose (see chapter 13).

I travel not to go anywhere, but to go.
—Robert Louis Stevenson

PRACTICE SUMMARY

The length of your practice while traveling will depend on your time available. Here is a summary of the Disturbed Rhythms series, along with some suggestions on using poses from the series in shorter sessions.

40 to 55 Minutes

POSE	TIME
Legs-Up-the-Wall Pose	4 to 7 minutes
Simple Supported Back Bend	2 to 3 minutes
Elevated Legs-Up-the-Wall Pose	5 to 9 minutes
Supported Bridge Pose	8 minutes
Supported Bound-Angle Pose	8 to 9 minutes
Supported Seated-Angle Pose	3 to 4 minutes
Basic Relaxation Pose with Legs Elevated	10 to 15 minutes

10 Minutes

POSE	TIME
Elevated Legs-Up-the-Wall Pose	10 minutes

20 Minutes

POSE	TIME
Elevated Legs-Up-the-Wall Pose	5 minutes
Supported Seated-Angle Pose	3 minutes
Basic Relaxation Pose with Legs Elevated	12 minutes

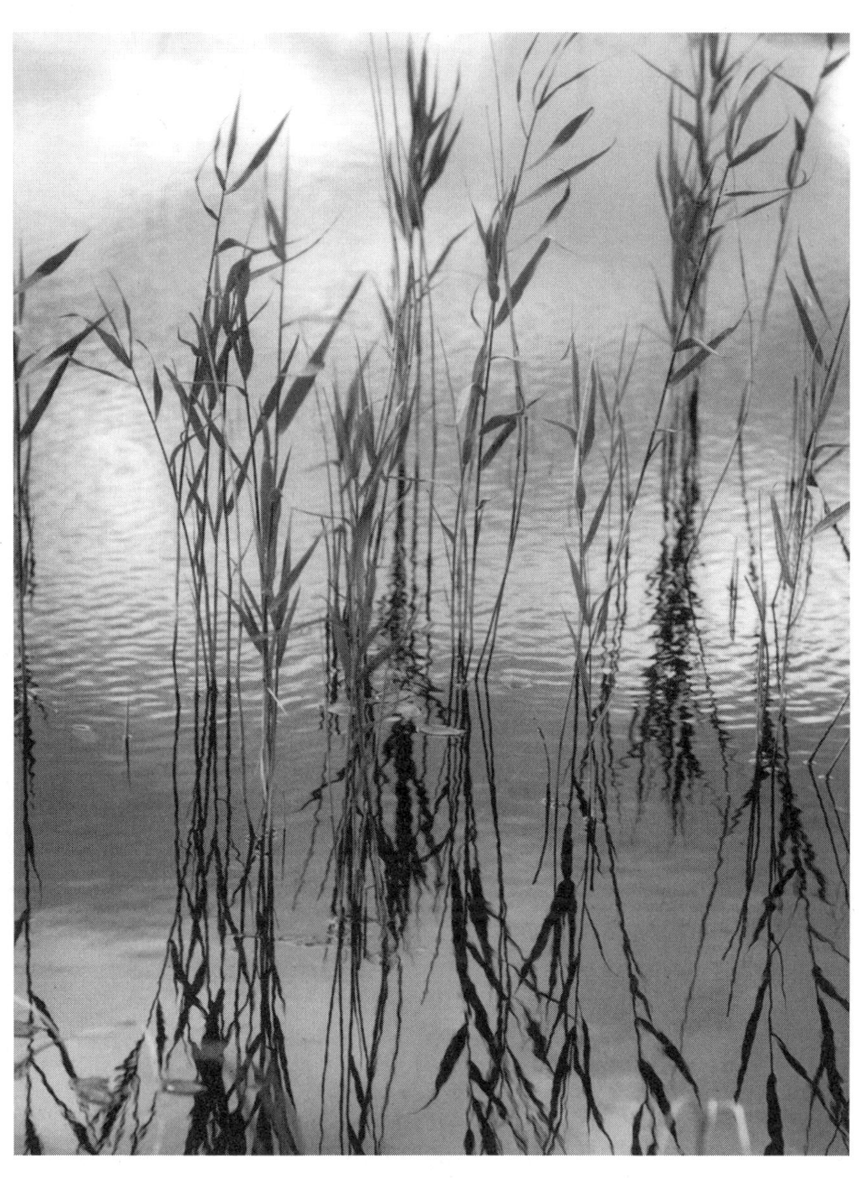

PART THREE: WOMEN'S WAYS

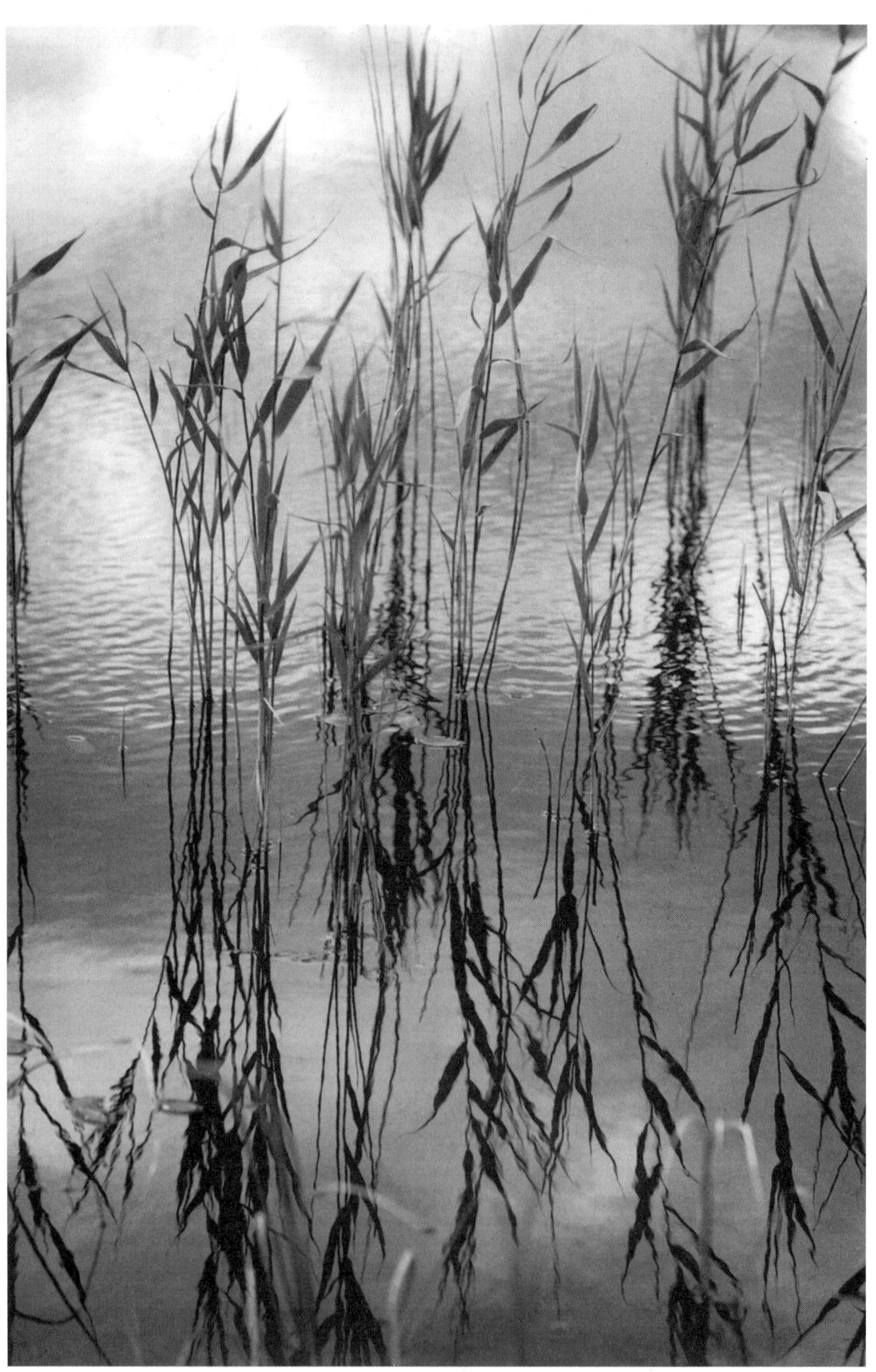

CHAPTER TWELVE

THE MOON CLUB

Honoring the Monthly Cycle

■ ■ ■

WOMEN TODAY are separated from the rhythms of nature more than at any other time in recorded history. Unlike the world of our foremothers, food is grown for us, plants are force-bloomed in hothouses, and air conditioning and central heating shield us from the elements. We leave no trace as we walk on ubiquitous cement pathways rather than on silky prairie grasses or sandy beaches. Nature has become something most of us only visit.

However, like our foremothers, we can turn to our bodies to experience our connection to nature. We have our monthly menstrual cycle to show us the way. Far from being a "curse," menstruation can be a quiet, reflective period—a time for each woman to honor the miracle of her body's potential for renewal.

I call the restorative series in this chapter the Moon Club, a name I gave several years ago to those women who attend my regular yoga classes and practice poses such as the ones in this series during the days of menstruation. I chose the name to reflect how the menstrual cycle unfolds in rhythm with the moon's passage from dark to full.

The Moon Club Series

The Moon Club series assists the body in releasing the menstrual flow, reducing fatigue, and moderating hormonal shifts. You can practice it throughout menstruation. Some women find it helpful to begin the series the day before bleeding begins. The Moon Club series may also be beneficial for premenstrual syndrome (PMS), endometriosis, and irregular periods.

The series consists of six restorative poses, designed to open the abdomen and alleviate cramps and lower back discomfort. It begins with an extroverted emphasis and moves to a more introverted one: supported back bends, followed by quiet forward bends, and ending with a variation of Basic Relaxation Pose. It takes about 20 minutes, but you can practice it for as long as 60 minutes. See the Practice Summary at the end of the chapter for suggested routines.

In general, a well-sequenced restorative yoga practice should include an inverted pose. However, women should not practice inverted poses during menstruation. A pose is considered inverted if the uterus, or lower abdominal region, is higher than the heart. Even poses that elevate the legs above the level of the heart should be avoided.

The rationale for avoiding inversions can be explained from both Eastern and Western perspectives. From the Western point of view, when the body is inverted, gravity causes those vessels supplying blood to the uterus to be partially blocked by the weight of the uterus dropping toward the floor. This may cause the menstrual flow to lessen or even stop for a brief time, perhaps a few hours, and then resume with a heavy flow. From the Eastern perspective, inverted poses block the *apana* energy from the pelvis with the same result. (See chapter 1 for a discussion of apana.) From either viewpoint, do practice the poses suggested in this chapter during menstruation, and save inversions for times other than Moon Club days.

Notice the effect of the Moon Club series on your menstrual flow during the hours after you practice. If the flow increases, or stops and then resumes, practice only Basic Relaxation Pose during the remaining days of this menstruation cycle. During your next menstruation, practice Basic Relaxation Pose and add one Moon Club pose per day. By slowly reintroducing the poses, your period should not be negatively affected. If it is, resume your practice of only Basic Relaxation Pose, and consult your health care professional before attempting other poses in the series.

> Your heart often knows things before your mind does.
> —Polly Adler

PMS, Endometriosis, and Irregular Menstruation

PMS is a constellation of symptoms that usually begin a few days before the onset of menstruation and extend through the first day or two of active bleeding. For some women, symptoms can begin as early as ovulation. While specific causes remain unclear, PMS is generally believed to be related to the hormonal changes preceding menstruation. Symptoms can range from mildly discomforting to severe in intensity, and include swelling and tenderness of the breasts, back pain, water retention, pelvic pain, food cravings, increased appetite, irritability, fatigue, headaches, moodiness, nervousness, and depression.

The human body is a wondrous thing.
—**Ralph Strauch**

If you experience PMS, the Moon Club series can help in two ways. First, it can reduce your physical discomfort. For example, poses that gently open the belly and hips can ease cramps. Stretches to the lower back may help with constipation and back pain. Second, practicing deep relaxation can help soothe the tension associated with PMS, and may even give you a little perspective on what you are feeling. Begin the Moon Club series as soon as you feel even the slightest symptom, and continue practice throughout menstruation.

Affecting five million women in this country, endometriosis is a condition in which pieces of the endometrium, or cells that line the uterus, embed themselves in other places of the body, primarily in the pelvic cavity.[1] This tissue is subject to the same cycle of swelling and shrinking as the endometrium within the uterus. Unlike the uterine lining, this tissue has no way to leave the body. What follows is internal bleeding, inflammation, and the formation of cysts and scar tissue. Intense pain may be experienced before or during menstruation, as well as during intercourse, urination, or evacuation of the bowels. Endometrial tissue that has attached to the back of the pelvis can cause lower back pain. In some cases, endometriosis leads to sterility.[2]

These poses cannot cure endometriosis. But if you have it, the Moon Club series can help you breathe and relax to relieve muscle spasm and pelvic congestion. Using the spreading, soaking, and squeezing principles described throughout this book, the Moon Club series opens and relaxes the uterus, abdomen, and lower back, which may have tightened in response to chronic pain. Practice the Moon Club series whenever you experience cramps or additional pain associated with endometriosis.

Menstruation can become irregular due to a wide variety of causes, including pregnancy, perimenopause, uterine fibroid tumors, illness, jet travel, stress, hormonal imbalances, excessive athletic activity, lactation, and hypothyroidism. When irregular, the body feels out of balance and especially vulnerable. If your menstruation is irregular, practice yoga regularly, with an emphasis on inversions and supported back bends. In addition, practice the Relax and Renew Series (see chapter 5) one day a week. When you do menstruate, practice the Moon Club series.

Irregular menstruation is also common as menopause approaches. If you are perimenopausal, practice the Moon Club series when you are menstruating. At other times, keep up your regular yoga practice, which should include an inverted pose. If you want to include restorative poses in your practice when not menstruating, use the Relax and Renew series (see chapter 5).

⁝⁝⁝ PRACTICE

Supported Bound-Angle Pose

Props

- bolster
- 4 long-roll blankets
- double-fold blanket
- belt or sandbag

Optional Props

- single-fold blanket
- eyebag
- extra blanket for warmth
- clock or timer

Supported Bound-Angle Pose is profoundly comforting and nourishing. Some of my students tell me it makes them feel cradled or held in a loving way. What better time is there to evoke these feelings than during menstruation or even a day or two before menstruation begins, especially if you are experiencing PMS?

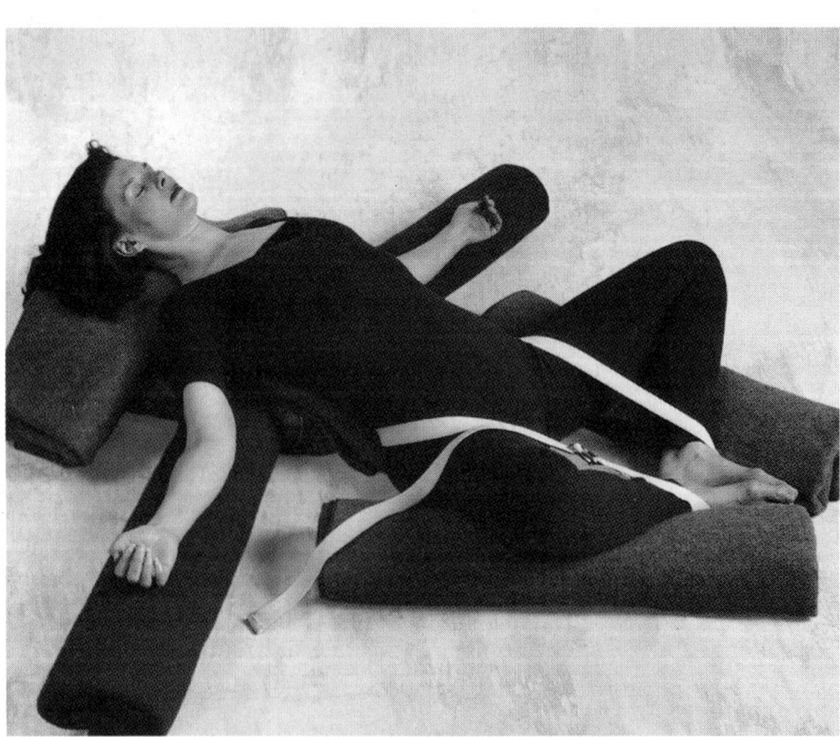

FIGURE 12.1
Supported Bound-Angle Pose

Setting Up. See page 34 for instructions on how to set up this pose. When arranging the long-roll blankets under your outer thighs, be sure to provide plenty of support to avoid sacroiliac pain. As discussed in chapter 16, the sacrum is the triangular-shaped bone of the spinal column, located just below the level of your waist. The sacrum joins the ilium bone of the pelvis and forms a joint called the sacroiliac joint. These bones are held together by ligaments. Because of hormonal changes during menstruation, these ligaments are especially vulnerable to injury and overstretching. In fact, some women are aware of the imminence of menstruation by the ache they feel in the area of the sacroiliac joint, as the ligaments loosen and stability of the joint is compromised.

In this unbelievable universe in which we live there are no absolutes. Even parallel lines, reaching into infinity, meet somewhere yonder.
—Pearl Buck

Being There. Supported Bound-Angle Pose is a wonderful pose in which to practice the Centering Breath: a slow, gentle inhalation, followed by a slow, gentle exhalation, followed by several normal cycles of breath, until you feel refreshed and ready to begin the Centering Breath again. (See pages 24 and 26 for a complete description of the Centering Breath.)

After a few rounds of Centering Breath with a focus on your lungs, bring your attention to your lower abdomen. As you inhale, keep your belly soft and receptive. Imagine that your breath penetrates the layers of your body—moving from the skin, to the muscles, to the organs. Let this inhalation bathe the uterus in relaxation. As you exhale, feel the diaphragm, lungs, ribs, and muscles of respiration contract, to press your breath out in a steady stream. Imagine that all congestion or discomfort in your lower abdomen is released on this stream. Let your breath return to its normal rhythm.

With your next Centering Breath, focus on the lower back. As you inhale, allow the back of the pelvis to receive the breath. As you exhale, let all tension in your lower back release on the steady stream of the breath. After each exhalation of the Centering Breath, take several cycles of normal inhalation and exhalation until you feel refreshed.

Repeat the Centering Breath for up to 10 rounds. Be sure to leave some time for several minutes of normal breathing before coming out of the pose.

Coming Back. Practice Supported Bound-Angle Pose for 5 to 15 minutes. Some women prefer to make this the focus of their Moon Club practice and stay in the pose up to 30 minutes. After relaxing so deeply, let the outside world come slowly into your awareness. Take in the sounds around you; pay attention to the sensations of your body.

As you feel ready, remove the eyebag, and slowly open your eyes. To come up, use the strength of your arms. Undo the belt or remove the sandbag from your feet. Straighten your legs, one at a time, to release any tension in the knees. Quietly move on to the next pose. If you are going on to your daily activities, take some transition time.

Benefits. Supported Bound-Angle Pose relaxes the abdomen and lower back, relieves cramps, and quiets the mind. Because it places the uterus in a semivertical position, it helps the menstrual flow move down and out. In other words, this pose harmonizes the apana, or feminine energy, in the abdomen by creating a receptive vessel in the belly and pelvis.

Caution

- See pages 35 and 36 for advice on this pose.

Reclining Crossed-Legs Pose

Props

- bolster
- 2 single-fold blankets
- 4 long-roll blankets

Optional Props

- standard-fold blanket
- 1 or more single-fold blankets
- eyebag
- extra blanket for warmth
- clock or timer

In the next pose in the Moon Club series, Reclining Crossed-Legs Pose, you sit on the floor with your legs crossed at the ankles and lean back onto a bolster and blankets. Even though Reclining Crossed-Legs Pose may be an unusual position for your body, the more care you take to position yourself and your props, the more comfortable you will be.

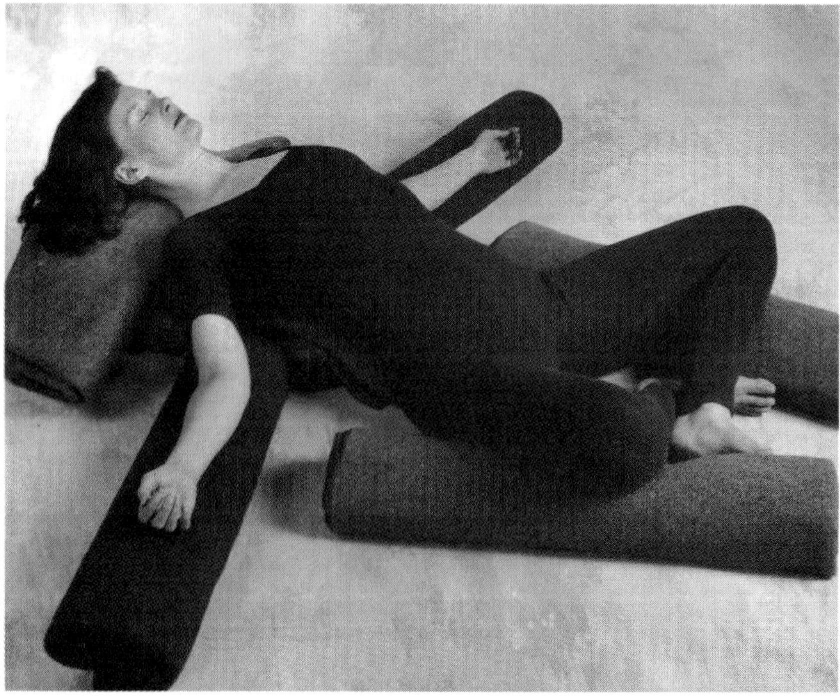

FIGURE 12.2
Reclining Crossed-Legs Pose

Remember, props are used to fit the pose to your needs. So often we experience stress by making ourselves try to fit the demands of our roles as employer, employee, parent, child, sibling, friend, or or partner. We seldom take the opportunity to slow down, breathe, and assess our needs. And if you are menstruating, life is even more demanding. Enjoy the next 5 to 10 minutes.

Feelings are untidy.
—Esther Hautzig

Setting Up. Sit in front of your bolster, with the short side next to your back. Place 1 or more single-fold blankets across the other end of the bolster to support the head, neck, and shoulders when you lie down. As always, experiment to find what feels best. For example, try 1 single-fold blanket and 1 standard-fold blanket under your head.

Place a long-roll blanket under each outer thigh to completely support the weight of your legs. *Use the long-roll blankets even if you are supple and open easily in this direction so you do not stress ligaments or the sacroiliac joint.* Make sure that your knees are equidistant from the floor. Remember, the point of the pose is not to stretch the inner thighs but to relax the abdomen and open the chest.

Cross your legs at the ankles. It does not matter which ankle is on top because you will change the cross halfway through the pose to balance the stretch. Lie back over the bolster, and rest your head, neck, and shoulders on the bolster and your arms on the single-fold blankets. You should feel some stretch in your chest and back but not discomfort. If your back is arched too much in this position or if you feel any strain in your knees, roll to one side and sit up. To alleviate back discomfort, place a single-fold blanket under your buttocks. (If you are using blankets instead of a bolster, reduce the number.)

Lie down again. Make sure that your head is well-supported. Your chin should be lower than your forehead. If you changed the height of the support under your back, adjust the support under your head and neck. Cover your eyes with an eyebag.

Being There. Rest on the props and let yourself feel completely supported. Swallow and relax your throat, jaw, and face. Breathe easily. Hold back nothing from letting go and relaxing.

As you relax, imagine a flower opening, petal by petal. Just as the flower opens, allow the cervix, located at the base of the uterus, to open to the menstrual flow. As you continue to relax, all cramping melts away. Trust that your body is in harmony with the deepest rhythms of nature.

After several minutes, change the cross of your ankles. It is not necessary to sit up to do this. Just make sure you practice for an equal time on both sides.

Coming Back. Practice Reclining Crossed-Legs Pose for 3 to 10 minutes. When you feel ready, take several deep breaths. Uncover your eyes. Slowly straighten your legs, one at a time. Roll to one side. When you feel ready, use the strength of your arms to sit up. Sit quietly for a few breaths.

Benefits. Reclining Crossed-Legs Pose softens the belly and relieves uterine congestion. During menstruation, the uterus fills with fluid. As it relaxes in this pose, the engorged organ can release the menstrual blood.

Cautions

- As in all restorative poses, you should not feel any pain or discomfort in your back. Take time to adjust your props. If you still experience pain, practice for half the amount of time the next time or skip this pose for now.
- If you feel pain or discomfort in your knees, adjust the height or placement of the long-roll blanket under each outer thigh. If the pain or discomfort persists, skip this pose for now.

Supported Forward Bound-Angle Pose

Props

- bolster
- 2 long-roll blankets

Optional Props

- 1 to 2 single-fold blankets
- chair
- towel
- eyebag
- extra blanket for warmth
- clock or timer

Based on the classic Bound-Angle Pose, this restorative variation is practiced here as a forward bend. The two previous poses in the Moon Club series are back bends, which open the heart and belly and free the breath. Forward bends express the feminine aspect of yoga, inviting us to move inward, away from our busy outer life of schedules and commitments,

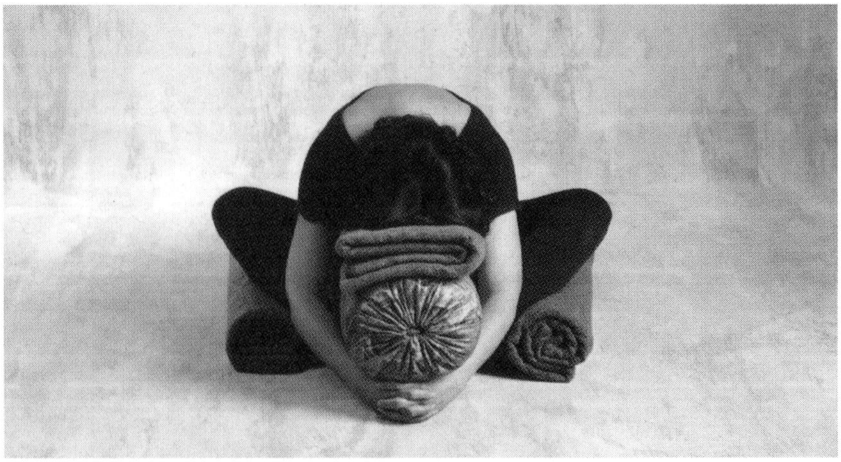

FIGURE 12.3
Supported Forward Bound-Angle Pose

to a rich inner life of quiet and solitude. They remind us to look inward for our strength and insights.

Setting Up. Sit on the floor. Position the bolster in front of you, with one end facing you. Place the soles of your feet together, and let your knees drop to the sides. Check your posture: if your lower back rounds, your chest drops, and your head thrusts forward, sit on the firm fold of the corner of 2 stacked single-fold blankets. The lift under your sitting bones will tip your pelvis slightly forward, so that your spine can lengthen and your chest and belly can open.

To the quiet mind all things are possible.
—Meister Eckhart

Place a long-roll blanket under each outer thigh, as you did in the previous poses. Lean forward and rest your torso and folded arms on the bolster. Do not force yourself to reach the bolster; imagine that the bolster is coming to meet you. If you feel any strain, place single-fold blankets on the bolster to raise the height of the support. If you need still more height, replace the bolster with a chair, and practice with your arms and forehead resting on the seat. You can place a towel over the edge of the seat if it feels cold or hard. You should feel completely relaxed and comfortable. For some women, however, the sacroiliac joint is aggravated even after making these adjustments.

Sacroiliac aggravation is experienced as a circle of pain about the size of a quarter or fifty-cent piece over the left or right side of the sacrum. You can locate the site of the joint by finding the bony prominence just to either side of the sacrum. If you feel any pain or discomfort in your back, you may find relief by adjusting your body asymmetrically to the bolster or chair. Slightly twist your body to one side and lean forward again. If this aggravates the pain instead of relieving it, then twist slightly to the other side. If neither adjustment helps, skip this pose and seek the advice of your health care professional regarding your sacroiliac alignment. Remember, yoga is not intended to overstretch or aggravate your musculoskeletal system. Pay attention to the alignment of your body in these poses, and be willing to shorten the time or skip the pose until your condition improves.

If you are able to proceed, keep your neck in a neutral position. Place an eyebag across the back of your neck and close your eyes.

Being There. Lean with complete trust onto the bolster or chair. Feel the gentle movement of your back as you inhale and exhale. Notice how the back ribs expand sideways and back to make room for the breath. Allow your body to assume its own natural breathing rhythm, and relax as layer after layer of tension melts away. Let this subtle process remind you to listen to your body's quiet messages during your daily activities.

Some women find that as they practice this pose, the body stretches and the props seem too high. If you experience this, slowly sit up and reduce the height. After adjusting the props, come forward again on an exhalation.

Coming Back. Practice Supported Forward Bound-Angle Pose for 3 to 5 minutes. Gradually increase your time to 10 minutes, as long as you experience no discomfort in your neck and lower back. When you are ready to come out of the pose, open your eyes and take several deep breaths. Lift your head slightly, and place your hands on the bolster, blankets, or chair seat. Press your hands down to help you sit up. Let the eyebag fall away from your neck. Place your hands under your outer knees. Slowly bring your knees together, with the help of your hands. Lie on your back, knees bent and feet on the floor. Remain in this position for several breaths. When you feel ready, roll to one side and slowly sit up.

Benefits. Supported Forward Bound-Angle Pose quiets the lower abdomen and relieves menstrual cramps. In addition, it gently stretches the lower back, an area that often tightens during menstruation.

Cautions

- If you feel pain or discomfort in your knees, adjust the height or placement of the long-roll blanket under your outer thighs, or move your feet farther away from your body.
- You should not feel any sacroiliac pain or discomfort. If you do, try the adjustments described in Setting Up, or skip the pose for now.
- If you experience any neck pain or discomfort during or after the pose, make sure that your neck does not sag during practice.

Do not practice this pose:

- if you have diagnosed disc disease in your lower back, or if you have spondylolisthesis or spondylolysis.

To be entirely at leisure for
one day is to be an immortal.
—Chinese Proverb

Supported Seated-Angle Pose

Another forward bend, Supported Seated-Angle Pose opens the legs out to the sides, like a dancer's warming-up movement before a performance. It is also common to women during childbirth and sexual intercourse. Signaling receptivity, this pose is one of the most feminine movements in yoga, especially when practiced with support. It is given here to relax the inner thighs, pelvic floor, lower abdomen, and uterus.

Prop

- bolster

Optional Props

- chair
- 1 or more single-fold blankets
- towel
- extra blanket for warmth
- clock or timer

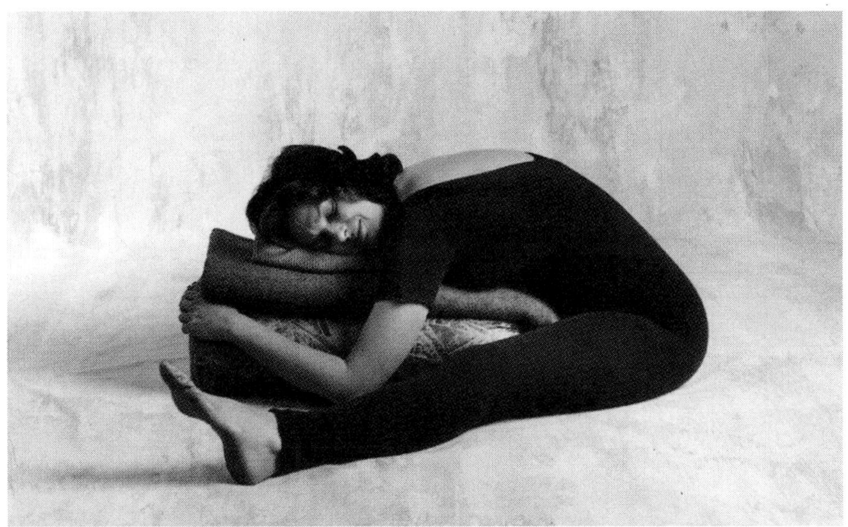

FIGURE 12.4 Supported Seated-Angle Pose

Setting Up. See page 46 for complete instructions on how to set up this pose.

Being There. Feel your legs supported by the floor and your torso supported by the bolster or chair. Notice the easy rise and fall of your breath. Allow your breath to fill the back of your torso, and release all tension in your lower back. Rest in the stillness of the present moment—poised between the open feeling in the belly and hips and the quiet feeling in the chest, eyes, and brain.

Coming Back. Practice Supported Seated-Angle Pose for 3 to 5 minutes, and gradually increase your time. If you are more experienced, you can stay up to 10 minutes. When you feel ready, open your eyes and rest for a few breaths. Place your hands on the bolster or chair, and use the strength of your arms to slowly sit up. Place your hands behind you and lean back to relieve your back.

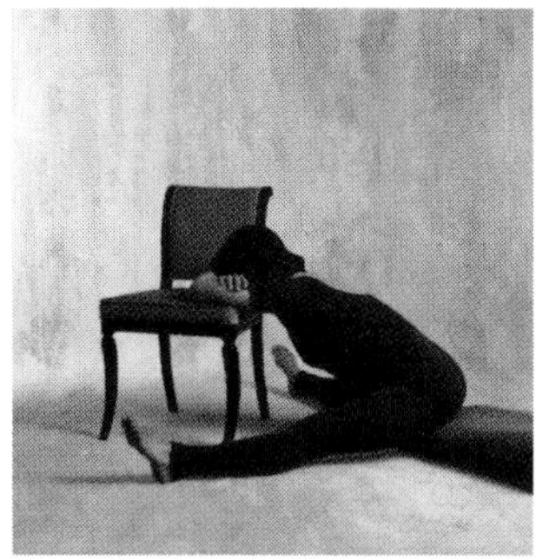

FIGURE 12.5
Supported Seated-Angle Pose, Variation

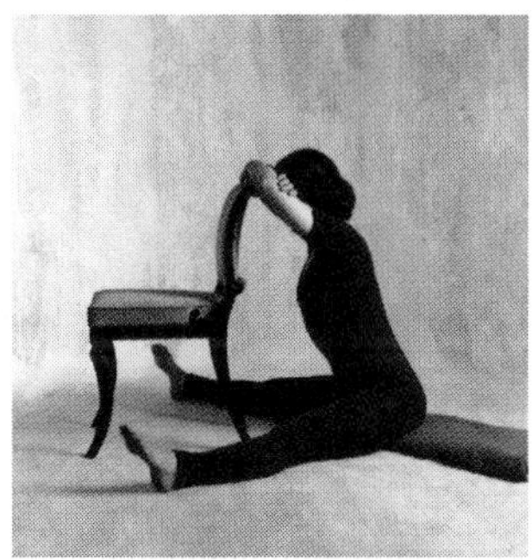

FIGURE 12.6
Supported Seated-Angle Pose, Variation

Benefits. Supported Seated-Angle Pose reduces nervous tension and relieves cramps. In addition, it opens the belly and relaxes the abdominal wall and uterus. By tipping the uterus forward and away from the spine, as well as up and out of the pelvis, the pose frees the uterus from being pressed on by the weight of the other organs. This action decreases the congestion in the uterus.

Caution

- See page 48 for more advice on this pose.

Supported Child's Pose

Prop

- bolster

Optional Props

- 1 or more single-fold blankets
- 2 towels
- sandbag
- long-roll blanket
- extra blanket for warmth
- clock or timer

We practice Supported Child's Pose during Moon Club days to benefit from the healing potential of turning inward. As we curl up, close our eyes, and press ourselves against the earth, we express the simplicity and innocence of a child at rest.

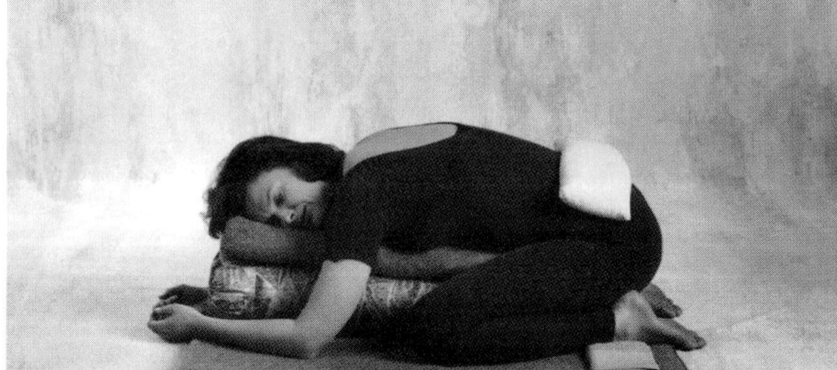

FIGURE 12.7
Supported Child's Pose

Setting Up. Refer to page 58 for complete instructions on setting up this pose. To enhance relaxation, practice with a sandbag on your lower back. To position it, hold the sandbag against your lower back as you bend forward. The weight of the bag helps to relax the muscles of the lower back and can reduce menstrual cramps.

Being There. Take several slow breaths. As you do, allow yourself to relax and receive the support of the bolster. Move your shoulders away from the ears. Allow your tailbone to drop toward the floor. Let your belly relax and feel supported. The pressure of the bolster against your belly may feel especially good if you have menstrual cramps.

Coming Back. Practice Supported Child's Pose for 1 to 5 minutes. Be sure to spend an equal time with your head turned in both directions. Open your eyes, turn your palms down, and place them on the floor under your shoulders. Press your hands into the floor, inhale, and sit up slowly onto your heels. Rest for a moment. Come to a kneeling position and immediately bring one leg forward, placing your foot on the floor. Press your hands on the forward thigh, and inhale deeply as you come to a standing position. Coming out of the pose in this way prevents discomfort in the knees.

Benefits. Supported Child's Pose relieves menstrual cramps and eases tension in the uterus. In addition, it gently stretches the lower back and quiets the mind.

Caution

- See page 59 for advice on this pose.

Basic Relaxation Pose with Calves Supported

Last in the Moon Club Series, this variation of Basic Relaxation Pose relieves discomfort in the lower back and lower legs. Do not place weight on the abdomen or elevate the legs more than 4 to 6 inches during menstruation.

Props

- standard-fold blanket
- 2 single-fold blankets

Optional Props

- sandbag
- extra blanket for warmth
- eyebag
- clock or timer

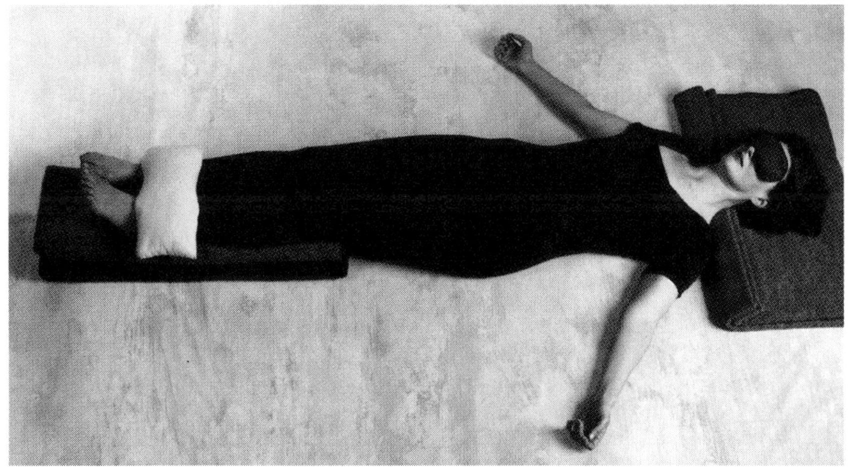

FIGURE 12.8
Basic Relaxation Pose with Calves Supported

Setting Up. See page 25 for a complete description of Basic Relaxation Pose. As always, before you lie down, position a standard-fold blanket on which to rest your head and neck. In other poses, blankets and bolsters have been placed at 90 degrees to your lower legs. In this variation, a stack of 2 single-fold blankets is turned lengthwise to support your calves. Place a sandbag across your ankles to anchor your legs on the blankets. Use the strength and support of your arms to help you lie back.

Being There. Practice up to 10 rounds of the Centering Breath. For guidance in this breathing awareness practice, see pages 24 and 26. When you have completed the Centering Breath practice, let your breathing return to its normal rhythm.

Coming Back. Practice Basic Relaxation Pose with Calves Supported for 5 to 20 minutes. To come out, slide your legs out from under the sandbag. Slowly bend one knee, then the other, and roll onto your side. Let the eyebag fall off by itself. Gradually open your eyes. Rest in this position for a few breaths before standing up.

Benefits. Practicing this variation of Basic Relaxation Pose with Calves Supported helps to relieve tension in your abdomen, reduce swelling in your legs, and ease lower back discomfort and cramps, which often accompany menstruation.

Cautions

- Do not place any weight on your abdomen.
- Do not elevate your legs more than 4 to 6 inches.

A thousand-mile journey
is begun with a single step.
—CHINESE PROVERB

PRACTICE SUMMARY

The length of your practice may depend on time available and how you feel. Here is a summary of the Moon Club series, along with some suggestions on using poses from the series in shorter practice sessions.

20 to 60 Minutes

POSE	TIME
Supported Bound-Angle Pose	5 to 15 minutes
Reclining Crossed-Legs Pose	3 to 10 minutes
Supported Forward Bound-Angle Pose	3 to 5 minutes
Supported Seated-Angle Pose	3 to 5 minutes
Supported Child's Pose	1 to 5 minutes
Basic Relaxation Pose with Calves Supported	5 to 20 minutes

5 to 10 Minutes

POSE	TIME
Basic Relaxation Pose with Calves Supported	5 to 10 minutes

15 Minutes

POSE	TIME
Supported Bound-Angle Pose	7 minutes
Basic Relaxation Pose with Calves Supported	8 minutes

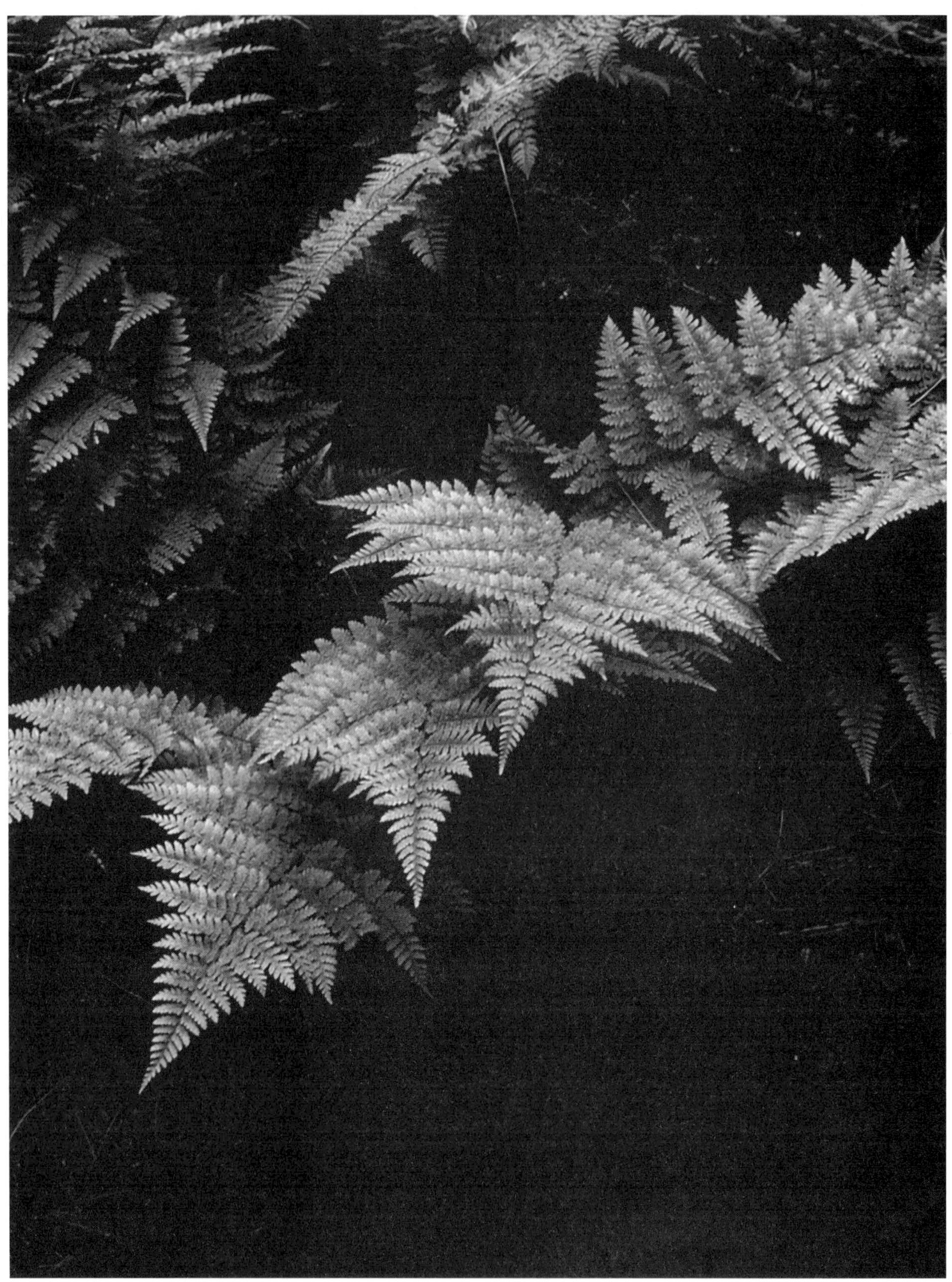

CHAPTER THIRTEEN

A PEA IN THE POD

Poses During Pregnancy

One of the most powerful and wondrous physical experiences a woman can have is being pregnant. Feeling life growing inside of you makes you profoundly aware of the complexity of nature and the intelligence of your body. Even though Western perceptions of the pregnant woman have changed over the generations, modern pressures still affect how you see yourself, your body, and your pregnancy. In the era of our foremothers, a woman stayed home and out of sight when she began "to show." Today's pregnant woman works, runs races, and plays tennis.

One thing is constant: The physiological and emotional changes that occur during pregnancy are potent. Pregnancy calls on a woman to relinquish her expectations of how things should be. One day you feel nauseous, the next day energetic. Pregnancy reminds you how important it is to care for your well-being. For most women, increased concern about good nutrition, sensible exercise, and adequate rest is a natural result of being pregnant.

Somewhere between the polarities of staying out of sight and overdoing is a middle path, one that celebrates your body's potential for carrying life. Each woman has to find this balance for herself. Many women find restorative yoga an opportunity to explore this middle path. These yoga poses can help throughout pregnancy and prepare for childbirth, both physically and emotionally. In addition, they can help you adjust to the postpartum period and to the demands of motherhood itself.

The Pea in the Pod Series

I got wings.
You got wings.
All God's children got wings.
—Negro Spiritual

This series is a sequence of six restorative poses that take you from standing, to sitting, to lying down. It begins with a modified forward bend, followed by a supine twist. Three supported seated poses come next. The series concludes with a Side-Lying Relaxation Pose, a variation of Basic Relaxation Pose. It takes about 20 minutes, but you can practice for as long as 80 minutes. See the Practice Summary at the end of the chapter for suggested routines.

This series benefits the healthy pregnant woman in several ways. First, it reduces general fatigue. By roughly the eleventh week of pregnancy, women are tired because they spend less time in the deeper, restorative stages of sleep.[1] Second, the series relieves back strain and fatigue from the increased demand of supporting the pregnant abdomen. Finally, some of the poses gently stretch the inner thigh muscles to help prepare for birth. Spending time each day practicing the Pea in the Pod series is excellent preparation for labor. These techniques are a natural complement to the childbirth methods taught today. Most of my pregnant students who have practiced the Pea in the Pod series continue it into the postpartum period, until lochia, the blood flow after childbirth, stops, and they feel ready to resume their regular yoga practice.

This series can also relieve other problems during pregnancy: morning sickness, high blood pressure, insomnia, and water retention. Specifics are listed under the Benefits section for each pose.

If you have had an abortion, miscarriage, or stillborn birth, practice the Moon Club series (see chapter 12). While designed for menstruation, the Moon Club series can be helpful until the lochia ceases, which is usually a matter of several days or perhaps a few weeks after pregnancy ends. Then practice the Relax and Renew series (see chapter 5) until menstruation resumes. Once your menstrual cycle is reestablished, practice the Moon Club series during menstruation, and follow a regular yoga practice at other times.

Important Reminders

Show this book to your health care professional before beginning this or any other exercise program, especially if there are any complications with your pregnancy, even though the Pea in the Pod series is usually appropriate at any stage of pregnancy.

Discontinue practicing any of the poses if they feel uncomfortable or disquieting, and then consult your health care professional and qualified yoga teacher about the appropriateness of the pose for you. If you are unable to get guidance, skip the pose for now. Try practicing it later in your pregnancy to determine if the changes in your body have made the pose more comfortable. If the difficulty arises late in your pregnancy, discontinue it until after the birth.

Avoid lying flat on your back after the first three months of pregnancy. When an expectant mother lies on her back, she can experience supine hypotension syndrome. In this position, the weight of the enlarged uterus, baby, amniotic fluid, and placenta falls backward and presses on the inferior vena cava. This is the major vein returning blood from the lower extremities and abdomen to the heart. Because veins can be compressed easily, this pressure can prevent blood from returning to the heart. This drops the output of the mother's heart on the next beat, lowering her blood pressure and decreasing the perfusion of blood and oxygen across the placental wall. The net effect is to reduce the amount of oxygen available to the baby.

Supine hypotension syndrome can lead to fetal distress. The mother's blood pressure may drop so low that she may actually feel faint. I can attest that this is a very strange sensation. All the poses presented in this chapter place the expectant mother in positions that avoid supine hypotension syndrome.

Avoid extreme stretching positions throughout pregnancy. You can practice active yoga poses or stretching exercises in moderation. However, this is not an advantageous time to push your limits. Because of hormonal changes during pregnancy, the connective tissue gives less support, and ligaments, which hold bone to bone, are looser. If the ligaments are overstretched, they can remain so after pregnancy. This lack of support can cause pain and discomfort. The Pea in the Pod series is designed to avoid this problem.

Familiarize yourself with chapters 1 through 4 before proceeding if you are new to this book and could not resist the temptation to turn immediately to this chapter. In addition, read the instructions for each pose in the Pea in the Pod series, including Cautions, before practicing.

If I didn't start painting,
I would have raised chickens.
—GRANDMA MOSES

Half Wall Hang

Prop

- wall or kitchen sink (or the side of a refrigerator or filing cabinet or a stable table or chair)

Half Wall Hang is a restorative pose that is easy to integrate into your daily activities. You can practice it several times a day—at home, at work, in airports, or whenever you need a rest. You can even invite a non-pregnant friend or your partner to join you in a moment of "social stretching." In this pose, you lean forward, using a wall or kitchen sink for support.

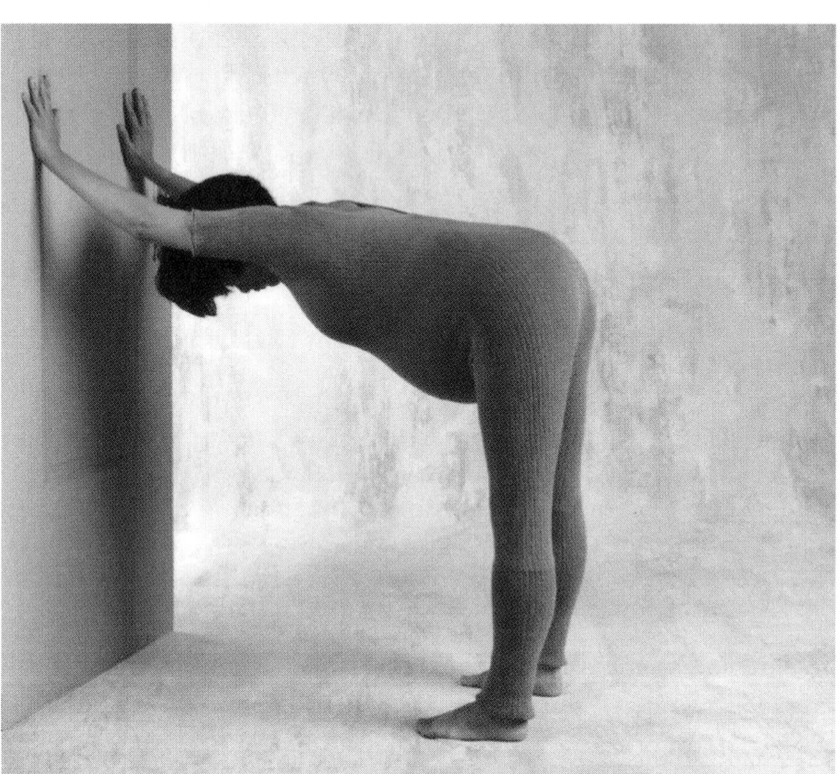

FIGURE 13.1
Half Wall Hang

Setting Up. If you are using the sink, grasp the edge with your hands, placing them shoulder-width apart or a little wider. Walk slowly backward, and bend forward, until your arms are straight and your spine is parallel to the floor. Your spine and legs should form a 90-degree angle.

If you are practicing at the wall, place your palms on the wall, at shoulder height and shoulder-width apart, or a little wider. Slide your hands down the wall as you slowly walk backward, until your arms are straight and your spine is parallel to the floor. If your back rounds, place your hands higher on the wall.

In either case, separate your feet approximately hip-width apart. This distance will increase as your belly grows. Make sure your feet are parallel, not turning in or out. Keep your legs straight, but be careful not to push back on your knees. If you tend to do so, bend your knees slightly and straighten your legs again, this time lifting your kneecaps and using your thigh muscles. Another technique to prevent pushing back on the knees is to move your feet farther away from the wall, so your weight is more on your hands and arms.

Being There. With your hands on the kitchen sink or wall, stretch away from the support. If you are at the sink, lightly lean back. Imagine there is increasingly more and more space between each of the bones of your spinal column. As you feel your shoulders open, let all your cares and worries fall away. Let your abdomen drop, and breathe slow, long, easy breaths.

Coming Back. Practice Half Wall Hang for 1 to 2 minutes. To come up, inhale deeply as you take a step toward the sink or wall and stand up. Be sure to inhale as you stand up to avoid getting dizzy.

Benefits. Half Wall Hang relieves tension in the back muscles. In addition, it moves the gravid (pregnant) uterus up and forward slightly, out of the pelvis, and away from the nerves on the back side of the body. Because gravity pulls the uterus down into the pelvic cavity, the uterus can press against a spinal nerve, causing pain to radiate down one leg. Half Wall Hang repositions the uterus and relieves this discomfort.

Half Wall Hang may relieve a cramp that pregnant women often experience in the round ligament that helps to hold the uterus in place. This ligament is the only one that contains contractile (muscle) fibers. All other ligaments are unable to contract; they can only be stretched.

A cramp in the round ligament is experienced as a sharp, stabbing pain on either side of the lower abdomen, just inside the hip bones. It usually occurs when you change positions rapidly, for example, rolling over in bed quickly to get up. As the result of sudden movement, there is a quick stretch to the muscle fibers of the ligament, which contract to protect against overstretching. Try Half Wall Hang to relieve this discomfort. This pose may also help to prevent the round ligament from cramping in the first place, so practice it several times a day. If this or any other pain is persistent, consult your health care professional.

Nothing, of course, begins at the time you think it did.
—Lillian Hellman

Cautions

- Remove your socks for this pose.
- You should not feel pain or discomfort in your back in Half Wall Hang.

If you do, try the following adjustments. First, make sure you are not overarching your back but are lengthening away from the sink or wall. If pain persists, come up and practice with your hands higher on a wall. If neither adjustment relieves the pain, skip the pose for now.

- If you feel any knee discomfort, make sure you are not hyperextending them. Lift up with the knees rather than pushing them back. You can also try the pose with your feet farther from the wall or sink.

Reclining Twist with a Bolster

Prop

- bolster

Optional Props

- single-fold blanket
- extra blanket for warmth
- clock or timer

The effects of the extra weight of pregnancy are compounded because of its position in front of the spinal column. Try this experiment: Pick up a medium-sized book and hold it close to your body. Then hold the book out at arm's length. Notice how much heavier the book feels when it is held farther away from your body. The same is true in pregnancy. As your pregnancy advances, the weight of your abdomen pulls on the supporting ligaments and muscles of the spinal column. Reclining Twist with a Bolster relieves the back discomfort associated with this extra weight.

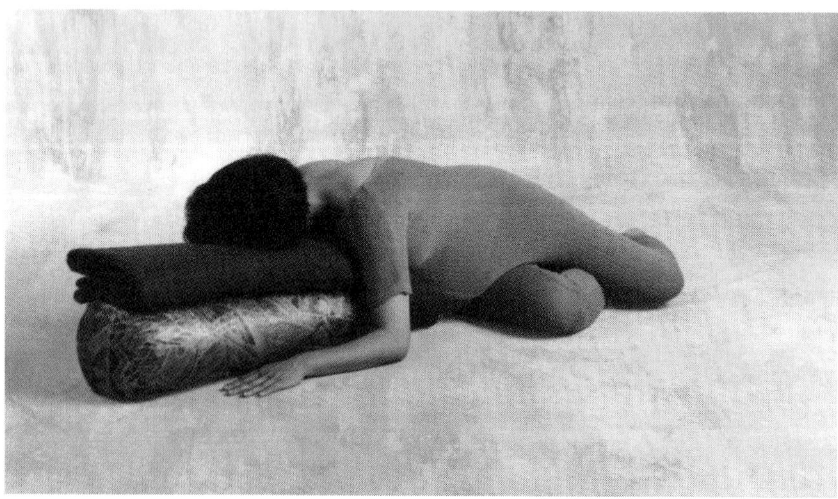

FIGURE 13.2
Reclining Twist with a Bolster

Setting Up. See page 44 for details on setting up this pose.

Being There. Relax the space between your shoulder blades. Use each exhalation as a reminder to release into the twist. Trust that you and the baby are completely supported by the bolster. Remember, as your pregnancy advances, you must make allowance for the size of your belly. In the first half of pregnancy, you may be able to twist farther than in the later stages. As your shape changes, be gentle with the twist—let most of it come in the upper back and shoulders.

Coming Back. Practice Reclining Twist with a Bolster for 30 seconds to 1½ minutes on each side. Your time in the pose depends on your comfort and level of experience. Do not be surprised if your experience on the second side is different from the first.

To come out of the pose, first turn your head toward your knees and rest for 1 or 2 breaths. Place your palms on the floor under your shoulders. Press down with your hands as you slowly sit up. Repeat the pose for an equal amount of time on the other side.

Benefits. Reclining Twist with a Bolster relieves stress on the back muscles and stretches the intercostals (the muscles between the ribs). As all the muscles relax, breathing is enhanced. In addition, the pose reduces water retention.

Cautions

- Follow the Coming Back instructions carefully to avoid straining your back and abdomen.
- You should not feel pressure on your abdomen when you come into or out of the pose, or while you are in the pose. If you do, increase the height of the bolster by adding a single-fold blanket. If you continue to feel the pressure, skip the pose for now.

Supported Reclining Pose

This is often the favorite restorative pose of my pregnant yoga students. For many, it has proven to be a good position during the early stages of labor. If you only have time for one pose in the Pea in the Pod series, try this one. While it requires many props and considerable setup time, it is well worth your effort. Be attentive to your needs throughout your pregnancy. Do not assume that the props that worked for you in the fourteenth week of pregnancy will work in the twenty-sixth week.

Setting Up. See page 103 for complete instructions on setting up this pose.

Props

- bolster
- 1 or more single-fold blankets
- 1 or more standard-fold blankets
- 3 long-roll blankets

Optional Props

- elastic bandage or eyebag
- extra blanket for warmth
- clock or timer

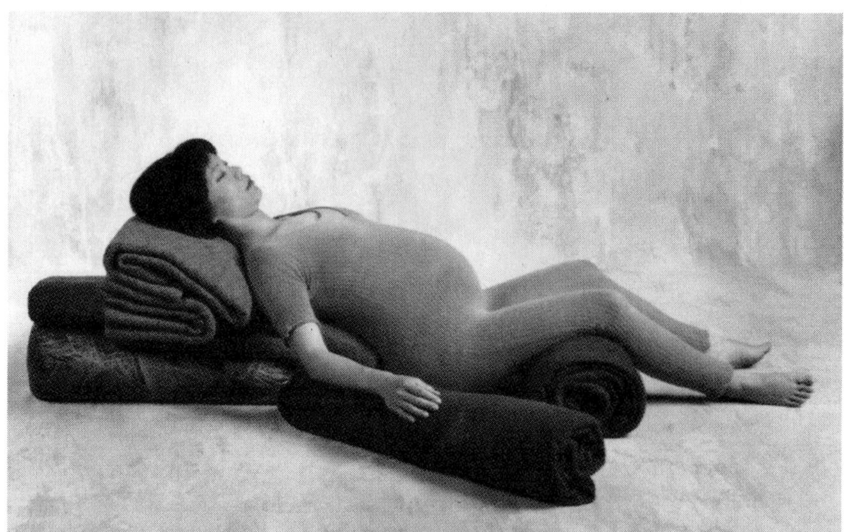

FIGURE 13.3
Supported Reclining Pose

Being There. Practice this pose in two phases. First, practice the Centering Breath. Second, focus on the baby.

Spend the first few minutes settling in. Breathe and feel your body completely supported by the props. When you feel ready, bring your attention to your breath. Begin the Centering Breath. (See pages 24 and 26 for guidance.) As you practice this breathing awareness technique, remember that your baby is inhibiting some of the movement of your diaphragm, so your long breaths might not be as long as your prepregnancy breaths. Practice the Centering Breath for up to 10 breaths. When done, let your breath return to its own natural rhythm.

When ready, move on to the second phase of practice. Because Supported Reclining Pose is so comfortable for most pregnant women, it is an excellent opportunity to focus on the baby. As you may have already experienced, it is when you are still that your baby begins to move. As you lie here, notice your baby's movements, however faint. Imagine that your baby is growing healthy and robust in your belly. Send feelings of love and acceptance to your baby and yourself. Appreciate yourself for your willingness to participate in one of life's greatest miracles. Relax and rest, knowing that all is well with you and your baby.

Coming Back. Practice Supported Reclining Pose for 5 to 20 minutes, depending on your comfort. It is virtually impossible to overdo this pose. When you are ready to come out, remove the eyebag, but keep your eyes closed. Let your eyes get used to the light coming through the lids before opening them. Bend your knees and use your feet to push away the knee support. Roll to one side and lie here for a few minutes before slowly sitting up.

Benefits. Supported Reclining Pose relieves nausea and enhances breathing. It is a gentle way to open the hips in preparation for childbirth. Because it is a gentle back bend, it can relieve tension between the shoulder blades. It is considered beneficial for the kidneys.

Cautions

- As I emphasized above, it is inadvisable to lie flat on your back during pregnancy. In this pose, the props should support you as if you were lying on a chaise lounge. It is also important that your chest lifts, so the top of the uterus, which in later pregnancy is high and near the breastbone, does not sink into the body.
- See page 105 for more advice on this pose.

Reclining Crossed-Legs Pose

In this pose, you sit on the floor with your legs crossed at the ankles, leaning back onto a bolster and blankets. Because the chest and lungs are opened and lifted, this position is especially good for practicing the Centering Breath. Some pregnant women can breathe in a more relaxed way in this position and find it helpful during the early stages of labor.

Setting Up. Refer to page 159 for a complete description of setting up this pose. Make sure you change the cross of your ankles and practice for an equal amount of time on both sides.

Props

- bolster
- 2 single-fold blankets
- 4 long-roll blankets

Optional Props

- standard-fold blanket
- 1 or more single-fold blankets
- eyebag
- extra blanket for warmth
- clock or timer

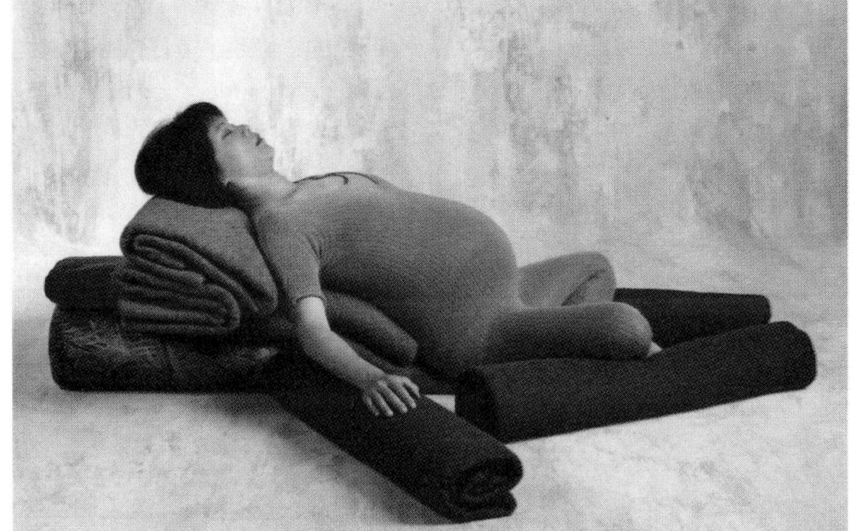

FIGURE 13.4
Reclining Crossed-Legs Pose

Being There. As always, spend the first few minutes settling into the pose. When you feel ready, begin the Centering Breath. (See pages 24 and 26 for more on the Centering Breath.) Follow the wavelike pattern of your breath. Let your inhalations and exhalations be rhythmic, fluid, and effortless.

When you feel your relaxation deepen, bring your practice of the Centering Breath to an end. Allow your breath to find its own rhythm. Be willing to be in the quiet space that lies just beneath your busy mind and busy life. These moments of deep relaxation are important for you and the baby. After the birth, so much will be asked of you that I encourage you to treasure these quiet, intimate moments. Just being present is the greatest gift you can give yourself and your baby.

Coming Back. Practice Reclining Crossed-Legs Pose for 5 to 15 minutes. Either roll to the side or use your arms to help you sit up slowly.

Benefits. Reclining Crossed-Legs Pose is helpful if you have a cold or are experiencing nasal congestion that comes with increased mucus production during pregnancy. It relieves mild nausea and headaches and benefits digestion and elimination. You can practice it during the early stages of labor.

Cautions

- As I emphasized above, it is inadvisable to lie flat on your back during pregnancy. In this pose, the props should support you as if you were lying on a chaise lounge.
- Pay particular attention to the comfort of your lower back, both in the pose and afterward. During pregnancy, hormonal changes loosen the ligaments that support the bones of your lower back, hips, and pelvis. You can avoid overstretch and strain with adequate propping. If you feel discomfort after your practice, stay in the pose for a shorter amount of time the next time.
- See page 160 for more advice on this pose.

Compassion directed to oneself is humility.
—Simone Weil

Reclining Heroine Pose

Reclining Heroine Pose is next in the series. In Sanskrit, this pose is called Virasana. The word *vira* is translated as "hero," "champion," or "warrior." Pregnancy, labor, and motherhood are a quest into the unknown, no less a challenge than those wondrous exploits undertaken by mythic heroes. I have renamed this pose Heroine Pose in recognition of the courageous journey that pregnancy and motherhood represents. Here we will practice the reclining variation. When I was pregnant, I practiced Reclining Heroine Pose in bed first thing in the morning to relieve nausea.

Props

- bolster
- 1 or more single-fold blankets
- 2 or more double- or single-fold blankets

Optional Props

- block, book, or blanket
- towel
- eyebag
- extra blanket for warmth
- clock or timer

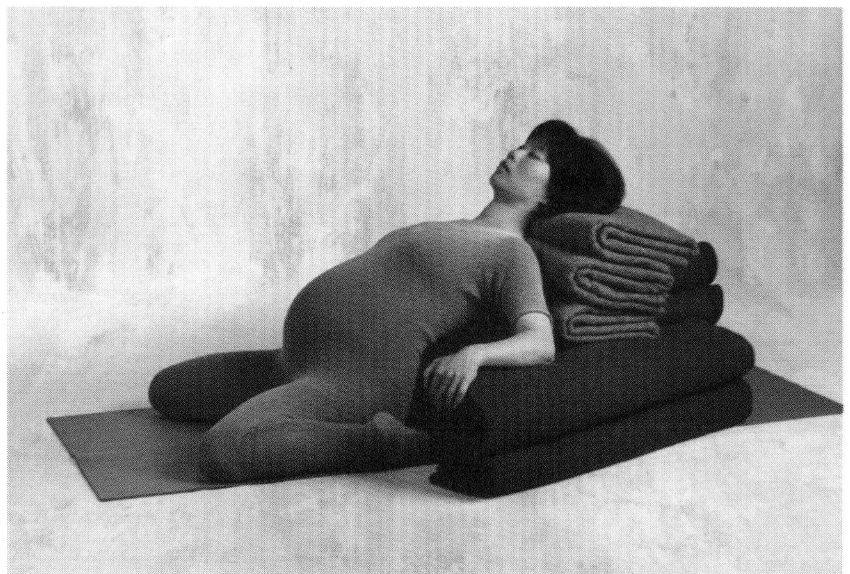

FIGURE 13.5
Reclining Heroine Pose

Setting Up. Before attempting the reclining variation of Reclining Heroine Pose, determine how comfortable you are in Hero Pose, the seated variation. Turn to page 128 for a complete discussion of Hero Pose, as well as instructions for setting up the restorative variation. Because you are pregnant, you will very likely need to modify the props throughout the forty weeks. For example, you may need to increase the prop height under your head or arms.

Reclining Heroine Pose is usually practiced with the knees together or nearly together, but most pregnant women find this uncomfortable. Let your legs open until your lower back, knees, and legs are comfortable, even if your knees are a foot or more apart. Cover your eyes with an eyebag. Place each forearm on 1 or more single- or double-fold blankets.

Being There. Lying with your hips, legs, and knees in this position may feel unusual at first, so give yourself time to get used to the sensation. Let the top of your thighs drop toward the floor.

Because your breathing in Reclining Heroine Pose is higher in the chest than in the previous pose, your abdomen will be a different shape. As you inhale, allow the top of your chest to expand horizontally. Maintain this openness as you exhale. When your legs feel heavy, your chest will feel lighter and expand more with each breath.

Coming Back. Practice Reclining Heroine Pose for 3 to 5 minutes. As you become more experienced, you can practice for up to 10 minutes.

There are two ways to come out of the pose. Option one: Use your arms to lift your torso up and forward, and come onto your hands and knees. Slowly straighten your legs, and walk your hands back toward your feet. Bend your knees slightly and stand up slowly. Option two: Use your arms to lift your torso up and forward, and come onto your hands and knees. Put one foot forward. With most of your weight on that foot, stand up as you bring the other foot forward.

Benefits. Reclining Heroine Pose relieves fatigue in the legs from walking and standing and helps to reduce swelling and varicose veins in the legs. It also relieves indigestion and nausea by lifting the diaphragm off the stomach and liver.

Cautions

- Do not practice Reclining Heroine Pose if you feel a sharp pull or pain in or around either knee. If you experience a generalized stretch or a slight ache that resolves itself immediately upon coming out or adjusting your props, it is probably fine to proceed. If difficulty persists, consult your health care professional.
- This pose may cause discomfort in the top of your feet, especially if you have high arches or tight shin muscles. Try practicing Reclining Heroine Pose on your bed.

It is only the first step
that is difficult.
—Marie de Vichy-Chamrond

Side-Lying Relaxation Pose

The last pose in the Pea in the Pod series is Side-Lying Relaxation Pose. Practice it as many times a day as possible, especially during the last few weeks of pregnancy when you are fatigued from carrying extra weight, or your sleep is disturbed by the baby's movements or frequent trips to the bathroom. Many women find this pose a helpful position during labor.

Props

- 3 or more single-fold blankets
- 1 or more pillows

Optional Props

- 2 towels
- bolster
- extra blanket for warmth
- clock or timer

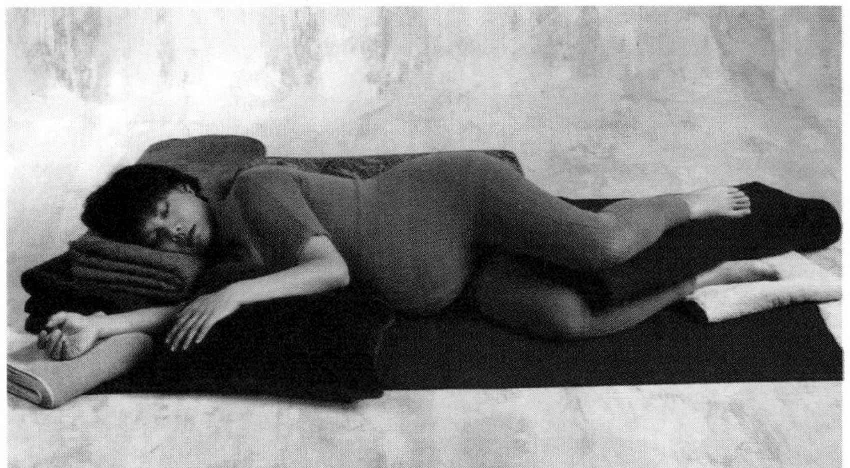

FIGURE 13.6
Side-Lying Relaxation Pose

Setting Up. Sit on the floor with your props nearby. Lean on one arm and lower yourself to the floor, so you are lying on your side with your knees bent. Place 1 or more single-fold blankets under your head and another between your knees. Place 1 or more pillows in front of you, and rest your arm on them. If you have a bolster, it feels reassuring to rest with it against your back.

For comfort, add a folded towel under the wrist of the arm you are lying on, and another under the ankle of the leg you are lying on. Make sure that your neck, spine, wrists, elbows, shoulders, hips, knees, and ankles are all gently flexed. Close your eyes.

Being There. Begin this variation of Basic Relaxation Pose by taking several slow and easy breaths. Swallow to relax your jaw, cheeks, and tongue. Let yourself rest completely on the floor and the props. This can be a very intimate time for you and your growing baby. Send feelings of love and acceptance to your child. Feel that you are cradling the baby and the props are cradling you. Know that you are safe, supported, and protected, as you rest and let go of everything but this precious moment.

Coming Back. Practice Side-Lying Relaxation Pose 5 to 40 minutes. If possible, let your own rhythms bring you out of the pose; for most women this occurs in approximately 20 minutes. Open your eyes and rest for a few more minutes. When you feel ready, use your arms to help you carefully sit up.

Benefits. Side-Lying Relaxation Pose relieves fatigue and insomnia and reduces high blood pressure. Many women find this side-lying a comfortable position for labor. Regular practice teaches relaxation skills that can aid labor.

Caution

- Pregnant women can practice Basic Relaxation Pose, described on page 25, during the first three months of pregnancy. After that, I recommend Side-Lying Relaxation Pose for reasons described above.

In our era the road to holiness
necessarily passes through
the world of action.
—Dag Hammarskjöld

PRACTICE SUMMARY

The length of your practice may depend on time available and how you feel. Here is a summary of the Pea in the Pod series, along with some suggestions on using poses from the series to practice for shorter periods of time.

20 to 80 Minutes

POSE	TIME
Half Wall Hang	1 to 2 minutes
Reclining Twist with a Bolster	1 to 3 minutes
Supported Reclining Pose	5 to 20 minutes
Reclining Crossed-Legs Pose	5 to 10 minutes
Reclining Heroine Pose	3 to 5 minutes
Side-Lying Relaxation Pose	5 to 40 minutes

10 Minutes

POSE	TIME
Side-Lying Relaxation Pose or	10 minutes
Supported Reclining Pose	

15 Minutes

POSE	TIME
Supported Reclining Pose	5 minutes
Side-Lying Relaxation Pose	10 minutes

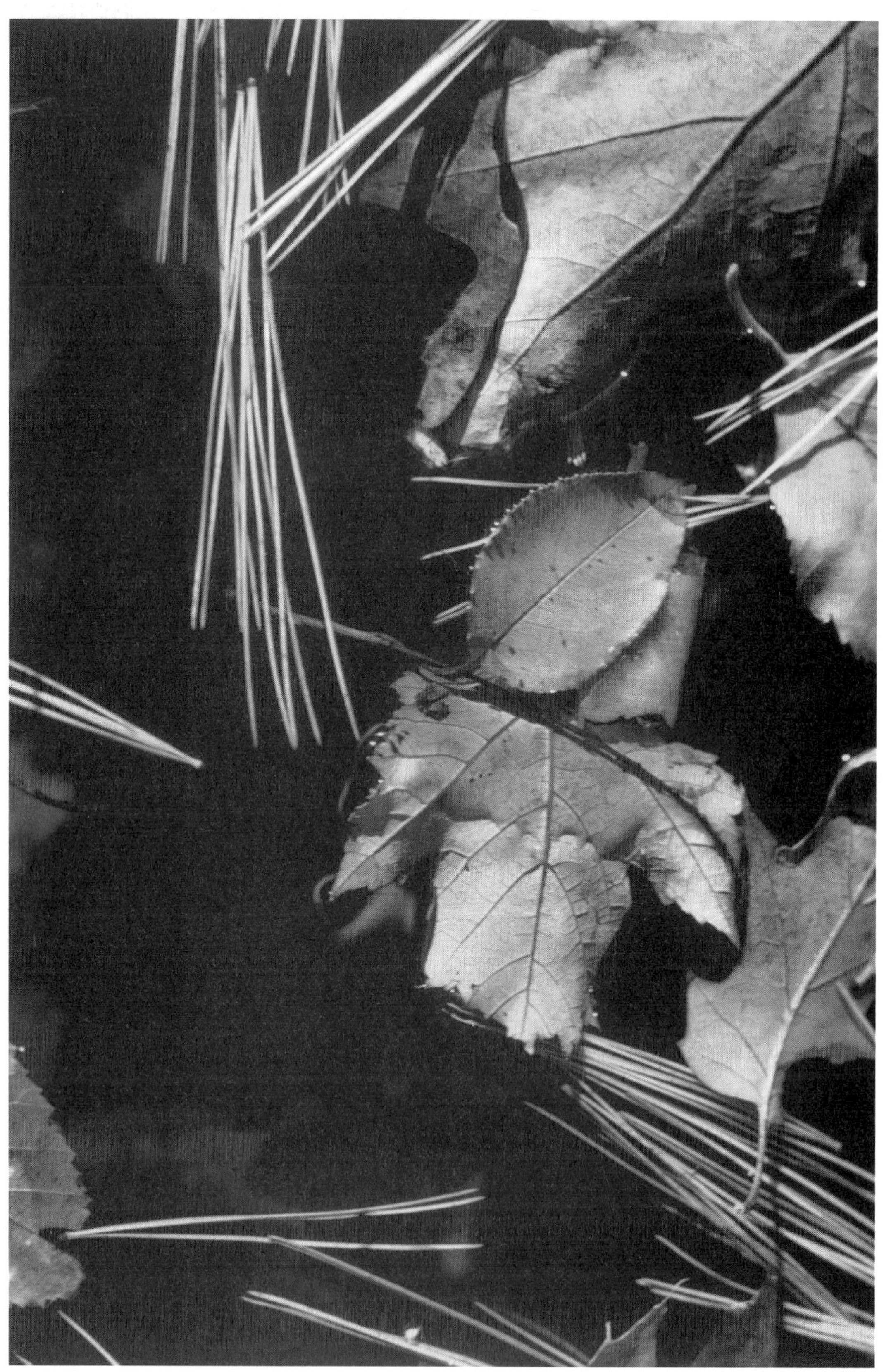

CHAPTER FOURTEEN

TRANSITIONS

Opening to Menopause

MENOPAUSE IS just as important a part of the heroine's journey as menstruation and pregnancy. But it has been misunderstood in our culture—not only by men, but also by women. Our health care professionals, educators, fathers, and most sadly our mothers and grandmothers taught us little, if anything, that was positive about this natural transition. "The change" was something to dread. None of us looked forward to living through years of unpredictable hot flashes, night sweats, insomnia, mood swings, headaches, depression, vaginal dryness, body odor, forgetfulness, and a limp libido.

Menopause is that rite of passage that marks the beginning of the second half of a woman's life. Just as menarche, the onset of the menstrual cycle, signals the passage from girl to woman, menopause heralds the passage to woman elder. The groundbreaking work of contemporary women—writers Gail Sheehy and Germaine Greer, doctors Sadja Greenwood and Susan Lark, psychologist Lonnie Barbach, to name only a few—beckons us to see menopause as a fertile time. In books, lectures, and workshops, women like these address how exercise, stress management, hormone replacement therapy and alternative therapies, attention to diet, and most important, women learning to trust their own experience can ease this transition. Like tribal elders, they tell us their stories and encourage us to tell our own. These women also model an empowering blend of sisterhood, compassion, expert advice, and common sense on which we and future generations of women can build.

What Is Menopause?

Technically menopause refers to a single event: the last menstrual period. The approximate two-to-five-year period during which we notice changes in menstruation and other symptoms is called perimenopause. During this time, the ovaries produce fewer and fewer eggs and gradually stop functioning, and ultimately menstruation ceases. Accompanying this is a gradual change in the production of hormones, including the estrogen group and progesterone. As these hormone levels drop, symptoms of perimenopause occur, usually between the ages of forty-eight and fifty-two. It can start as early as thirty-five and as late as sixty.

Some women transition easily; many have a rocky road; most have some of both. And perimenopause comes at a time when other stressful events are challenging women. Sick or dying parents or friends, career demands, a partner retiring or cutting back on work hours, changing financial status, and children leaving home do little to smooth the effects of the roller-coaster ride of changing hormone levels.

The Opening to Menopause Series

One must be able to let things happen.
—C.G. Jung

This chapter describes the Opening to Menopause series—eight restorative poses that stimulate the ovaries and pituitary gland to produce more hormones. The series begins with two modified forward bends, followed by a supported back bend. A reclining pose and two inverted poses come next. The series winds down with another forward bend and concludes with a variation of Basic Relaxation Pose. Ideally these poses should help you feel calmer, less fatigued, and less battered by your perimenopausal experiences. As always, restorative poses can help you be present to your own experience, rather than turning away from it.

This series takes from 60 to 80 minutes. See the Practice Summary at the end of the chapter for suggested shortened routines. I recommend that you alternate the Opening to Menopause series with the Moon Club series. When you are not menstruating, practice the menopause series three times a week; when you are, no matter how short or irregular, practice the menstruation series in chapter 12.

Twentieth-century anthropologist Margaret Mead wrote about "post-menopausal zest," that resurgence of energy that follows the shift in hormonal and reproductive states.[1] It is good to know there is light at the end of the tunnel. But I assert there is also light in the tunnel—in the fruitful darkness of menopause.

Wall Hang

A supported forward bend, Wall Hang reverses the position in which we usually hold the head, neck, and torso. As you rest your buttocks against the wall and come into a forward bend, the back muscles and backs of the legs release, and the mind quiets. By allowing your head to hang, the pituitary gland, located in the center of the brain, is stimulated. This head position may relieve some perimenopause symptoms.

Prop
- wall

Optional Props
- nonskid mat
- chair
- clock or timer

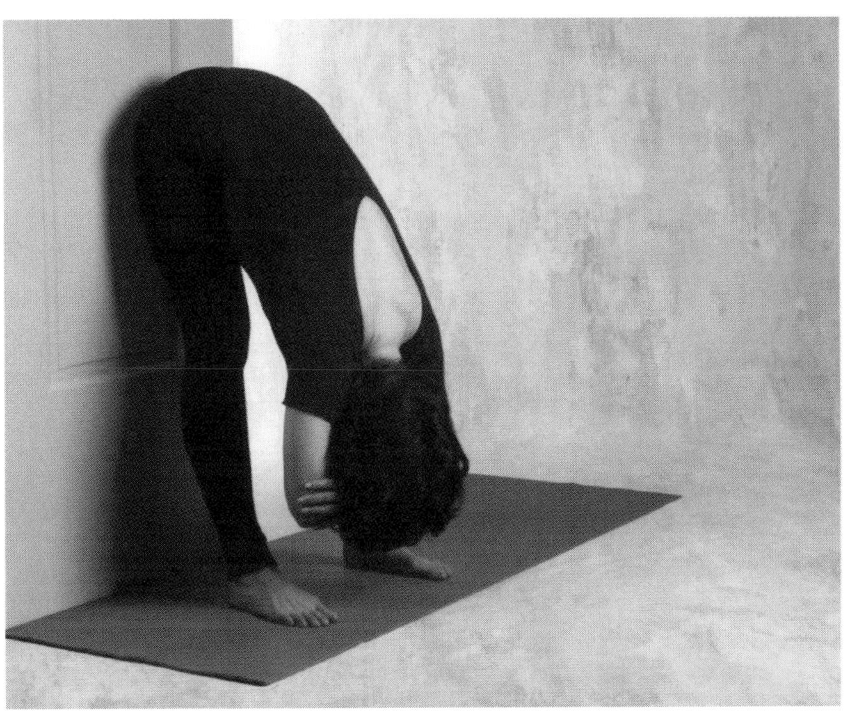

FIGURE 14.1 Wall Hang

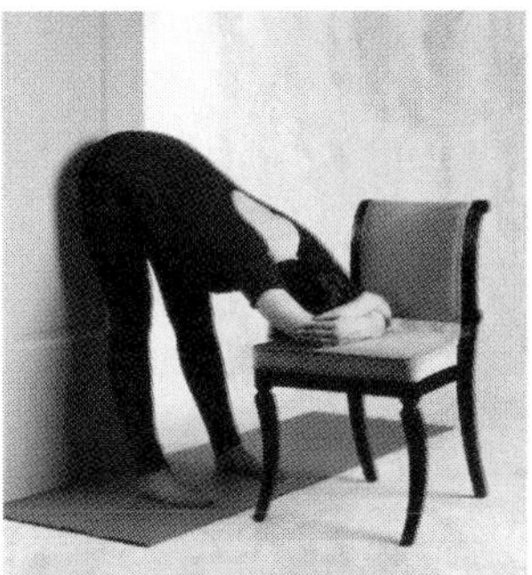

FIGURE 14.2
Wall Hang, Variation

Setting Up. Rest your buttocks against the wall, and walk your feet 12 to 16 inches forward. Separate your feet approximately 14 to 16 inches. Exhale as you bend forward. Fold your elbows and let the weight of the arms and torso gently pull you down. Let your head hang.

Keep your legs straight and your quadriceps, the muscles at the front of the thighs, active. When these muscles contract, the knee joints are stabilized. In addition, because of a physiological response called reciprocal innervation, when the quadriceps contract, there is a reflex release in the hamstrings, muscles located at the back of the thighs and opposing the quadriceps. The release of the hamstrings allows you to come forward in a way that protects your lower back.

Letting go a little improves life. Letting go a lot brings happiness and joy.
—Jim McGregor

To check if the quadriceps are active, try to move the kneecaps from side to side with your fingers. If the quadriceps are working, the kneecaps will stay firmly in place. If the kneecaps move easily, you will know that you are not using the power of the quadriceps muscle. If you can move your kneecaps easily, come up slowly as you inhale. Lean against the wall for a few seconds, especially if you feel dizzy. Remain against the wall for balance, and raise one leg about 18 inches from the floor, keeping it straight. Reach down and feel how strongly the quadricep is working. Lower your leg and try the same thing with your other leg. Resume Wall Hang, and recreate this same action in your quadriceps.

If tightness in your hamstrings prevents you from coming forward easily, practice Wall Hang with your hands resting on a chair seat, or substitute Half Wall Hang from chapter 13. Take heart: with practice of Half Wall Hang and other yoga poses, your hamstrings will loosen. Try Wall Hang occasionally to check your progress.

Being There. Feel your hamstrings stretch, as you release into Wall Hang. Relax your abdomen, as you breathe normally. Let your head hang between your folded arms. Gently move your head from side to side a few times, as if you were gesturing "no," to help relax your neck and shoulders. Allow your spine to lengthen, as all tension in your back drains away.

Coming Back. Practice Wall Hang for 30 seconds to 1 minute. As you become more experieced, you can stay as long as 2 minutes. To come out, place your hands on your legs. Inhale deeply (to avoid dizziness), as you walk your hands up your legs and come to standing. When you are fully upright, lean against the wall for several breaths, and notice the quieting effect the pose has had on your mind.

Benefits. Wall Hang is a modified inversion. Poses that place the head lower than most or all of the body stimulate the endocrine system, especially the pituitary gland, which controls the changes in hormone levels that occur in menopause. Remember, it is the withdrawal of estrogen and other hormones from the body that initiates perimenopause. The pose also places pressure on the abdomen and uterus, squeezing blood from the abdominal organs. When you come out of the pose, the organs are then soaked or bathed in fresh blood. This alternate squeezing and soaking enhances the functioning of the ovaries and the hormones they produce. Finally, Wall Hang soothes the nervous system and quiets the mind.

Cautions

- Remove your socks for this pose.
- Do not practice this pose if you have diagnosed disc disease in your lower back or neck, sacroiliac dysfunction, or radiating pain or tingling in one or both arms or legs. Practice Half Wall Hang from chapter 13 instead.

Hanging Dog Pose

Hanging Dog Pose is based on the classical Downward-Facing Dog Pose. Like Wall Hang, it is a modified inversion with many of the same hormonal effects. But this pose has an added benefit: it is also a gentle back bend that stretches the upper back and shoulders. Sometimes breast size increases during perimenopause. Hanging Dog Pose can help to relieve the postural strain created by heavy breasts.

Props

- nonskid mat
- belt
- door with doorknobs

Optional Props

- chair
- clock or timer

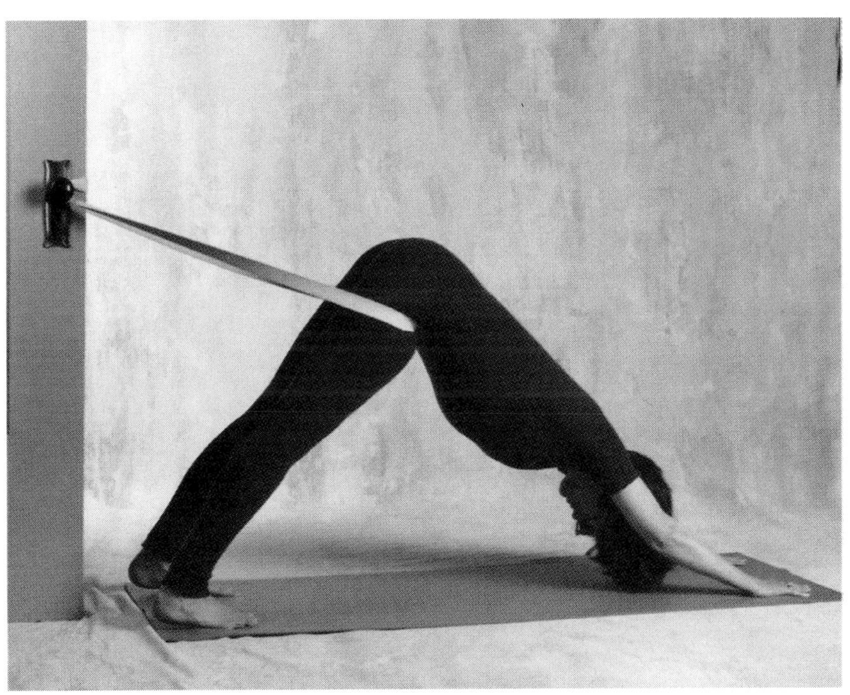

FIGURE 14.3 Hanging Dog Pose

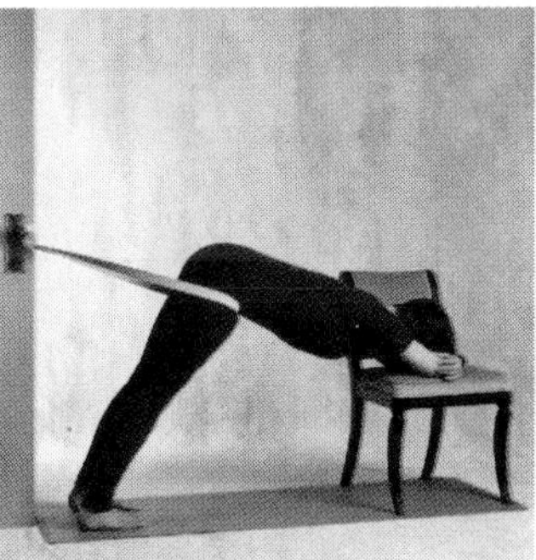

FIGURE 14.4
Hanging Dog Pose, Variation

Setting Up. See page 73 for instructions on setting up the pose.

Being There. Once you are in the inverted V position, feel your hands and feet in firm contact with the floor. All of your knuckles should touch the floor. Spread your thumbs away from your fingers. Make sure your ankles do not roll in or out but remain in a neutral position. Likewise, make sure your heels do not turn toward one another, but almost turn away from each other. Press the ball of your big toes firmly into the floor.

Take several deep breaths. Lengthen the muscles on either side of your spine. Soften your belly so it feels hollow, as you allow it to lift toward your spinal column. Relax your neck and drop your head. Feel your hands in contact with the floor. As the weight of your body moves back, your arms lift away from your hands, and your spine lifts away from your arms.

Enjoy this feeling of lightness.

Coming Back. Practice Hanging Dog Pose for 30 seconds to 1½ minutes. To come out, bend your knees and walk back with your hands to stand up. Remain still for a few moments and with your eyes open, take a few breaths before stepping out of the belt and continuing with your practice.

Benefits. A modified inversion, Hanging Dog Pose helps to stimulate the pituitary gland, which can positively effect its release of hormones, thereby easing the symptoms of perimenopause. It helps to increase the blood flow to your upper torso, head, and neck. This flow refreshes the muscles of your upper back and neck. In addition, the pose relieves muscle tightness in the lower back and shoulders from prolonged sitting, softens the abdomen, and quiets the mind.

Caution

- See page 74 for advice on this inverted pose.

Age seldom arrives smoothly or quickly. It's more often a succession of jerks.
—Jean Rhys

Mountain Brook Pose

The ocean is ever-changing, ever renewing. The waves advance and recede in a predictable rhythm. The water that rushed to shore an hour ago may be many miles out to sea in this moment. This rhythm is a powerful image for the woman in perimenopause. As the roles of young woman and baby maker recede, something new fills the space. Mountain Brook Pose is a way to explore this new space. Let your breath show you the way.

Props

- bolster
- 2 single-fold blankets
- long-roll blanket

Optional Props

- standard-fold blanket
- eyebag
- extra blanket for warmth
- clock or timer

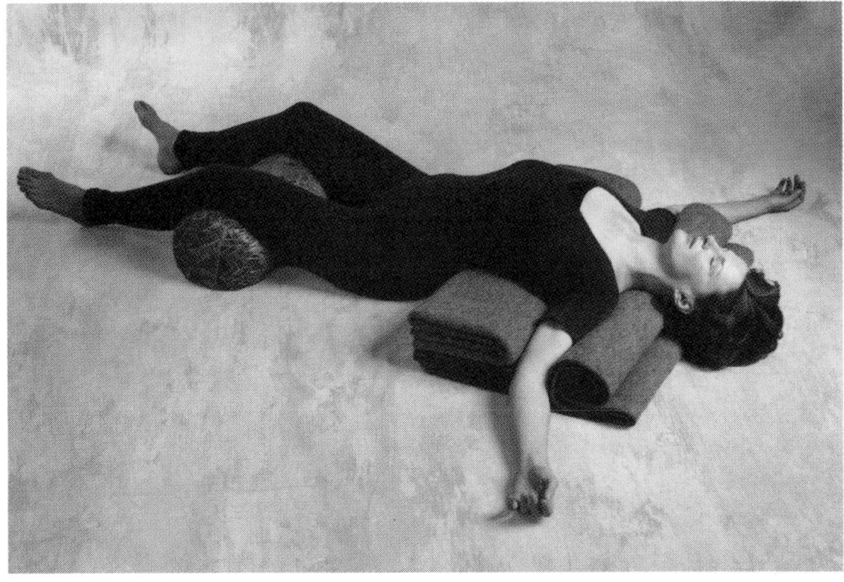

FIGURE 14.5
Mountain Brook Pose

Setting Up. See page 37 for instructions on setting up this pose.

Being There. As you breathe and feel the support of the props, gently bring your attention to your heart and arms. Receive whatever feelings arise from your heart. Imagine that the position of your arms allows you to embrace these feelings—even if they are ambiguous ones about your new place as a woman, freed from the sweet but difficult times of childbearing. Be gentle with yourself.

Coming Back. Practice Mountain Brook Pose for at least 5 minutes. If you are very comfortable or are an experienced yoga student, stay for as long as 15 minutes. To come out, remove the eyebag and use your hands to gently lift your head. Then slide off the props toward your head, using your arms. Let your legs rest over the bolster. Lie on the floor for a few minutes before rolling to one side and getting up.

Benefits. Because of the open position of the throat, Mountain Brook Pose has a regulating effect on the thyroid gland, including balancing energy and the tendency to gain weight during menopause. In addition, Mountain Brook Pose counteracts the slumped sitting posture that so many of our daily activities reinforce. It helps you breathe more fully, improves digestion, reduces fatigue, and can lift your mood if you feel down.

Caution

▸ See page 38 for more advice on this pose.

Supported Bound-Angle Pose

Props

- bolster
- 4 long-roll blankets
- double-fold blanket
- belt or sandbag

Optional Props

- single-fold blanket
- eyebag
- extra blanket for warmth
- clock or timer

You may have noticed that I include Supported Bound-Angle Pose in several sequences in this book. In my own yoga practice, I go back to it again and again—and for good reason. Women are experienced at caregiving. We care for the baby growing in the womb, for the newborn with breast milk, and with a watchful eye for the toddler. We extend this skill to family and friends. Important in caregiving is balance: the caregiver needs to be able to receive support from self and others. Supported Bound-

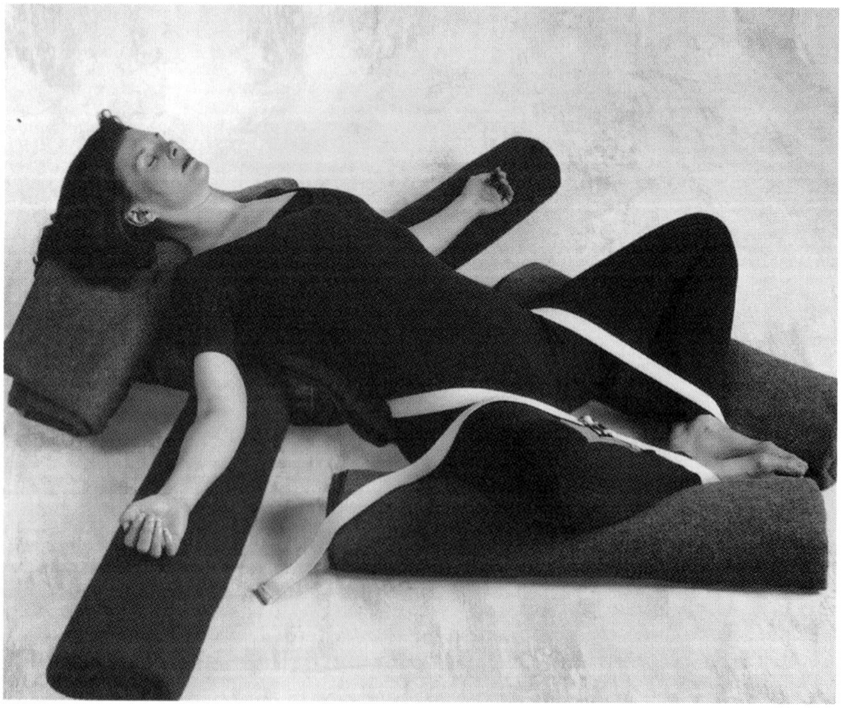

FIGURE 14.6
Supported Bound-Angle Pose

Angle Pose gives a woman a chance to turn this skill toward herself, which is particularly important during the challenging times of menopause.

Setting Up. See page 34 for instructions on setting up this pose.

Being There. As you settle into the pose, feel the pleasure of being completely supported. Your neck, arms, back, and legs are held by the props. Your belly, uterus, and ovaries are cradled by the pelvis. Notice the easy rise and fall of your breath.

Troubles, like babies, grow larger by nursing.
—Unknown

Because of the position of the lungs, this pose is good for practicing the Centering Breath: a slow, gentle inhalation, followed by a slow, gentle exhalation, followed by several normal cycles of breath, until you feel refreshed and ready to begin the Centering Breath again. (See pages 24 and 26 for guidance in this breathing awareness practice.) You can practice the Centering Breath for 10 breaths. When finished, allow your breath return to its natural rhythm, and rest on the props for the remainder of the the time.

Coming Back. Practice Supported Bound-Angle Pose for up to 15 minutes. After relaxing so deeply, let the outside world come slowly into your awareness. Take in the sounds around you; pay attention to the sensations of your body. Remove the eyebag and slowly open your eyes.

If you have back problems, come up by slipping your feet out from the belt or the sandbag, bringing your knees together, and carefully rolling to one side. Lie quietly for a few moments, and then use your arms to help you sit up.

If you do not have back problems, come up by pressing down with your arms and sitting up slowly. Undo the belt or remove the sandbag from your feet. Slowly stretch your legs out in front of you to release any tension in the knees. As you move through your day, remain secure in your connection to your body, trusting that the changes you are going through are a perfect part of your life.

Benefits. Supported Bound-Angle Pose places the abdomen, uterus, ovaries, and vagina in a position that frees these areas of constriction and tension that inhibit balanced hormonal activity. It helps to reduce the severity and duration of mood swings. In addition, those with high blood pressure, breathing problems (see chapter 10), and headaches (see chapter 8) often find this pose helpful.

Caution

- See pages 35 and 36 for advice on this pose.

Elevated Legs-Up-the-Wall Pose

Props

- bolster
- single-fold blanket

Optional Props

- eyebag
- towel
- double-fold blanket
- 1 or more single-fold blankets
- standard-fold blanket
- extra blanket for warmth
- clock or timer

Keeping a balanced perspective about life enables us to see clearly what is really important. Occasionally we lose our way, and it is helpful to consider something from a different viewpoint. Not only is Elevated Legs-Up-the-Wall Pose beneficial for the physical and emotional changes during menopause, but turning things upside down offers a good chance to consider the place of menopause in your life.

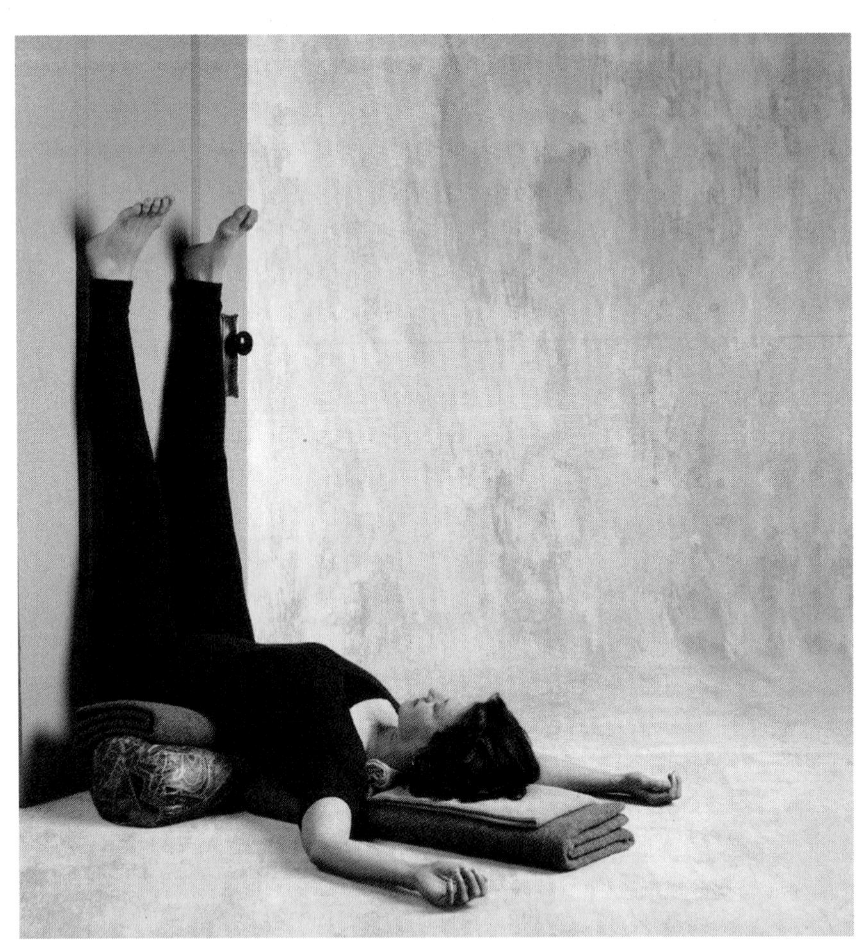

FIGURE 14.7
Elevated Legs-Up-the-Wall Pose

Setting Up. See page 41 for details on setting up this pose.

Being There. Let yourself be supported by the bolster and the floor. Forget the outside world for a few minutes; allow yourself the important task of doing nothing. Take slow and steady breaths. Because your chest is supported in an open position, you may experience a sense of release. Enjoy the sensation of fatigue draining from your legs, the opening of your back and shoulders, and the quieting of your mind. Let go of the impulse to change your position.

Coming Back. Practice Elevated-Legs-Up-the-Wall Pose for up to 15 minutes. To come out, remove the eyebag and bend your knees. Press your feet on the wall, and lift your pelvis slightly. Push the bolster toward the wall with your hands, and slide your body away from the wall by pressing with your feet. Lie on the floor for a few moments, with your lower legs supported by the bolster. Roll to the side and get up slowly.

Benefits. Elevated Legs-Up-the-Wall Pose allows blood and lymph to pool in the belly, which soaks the reproductive organs in oxygen. Forward bends, such as Wall Hang, Hanging Dog Pose, and Child's Pose, do the opposite, by squeezing fluids away from the reproductive organs. This alternate squeezing and soaking regulates the function of the reproductive organs during menopause.

In addition, this pose reduces the systemic effects of stress. It quiets the mind and refreshes the heart and lungs. It is beneficial for those who retain water and whose legs swell easily, and for those who have varicose veins or stand for long periods.

Cautions

- If you get pregnant during perimenopause, do not practice this pose past the third month. Do not practice it if you are at risk for miscarriage.
- See page 43 for more advice on this inverted pose.

There are only three kinds
of persons in the world:
the immovable,
the movable,
and those that move.
—**Persian Proverb**

Supported Bridge Pose

Props

- 2 bolsters

Optional Props

- 2 or more single-fold blankets
- eyebag
- towel
- extra blanket for warmth
- clock or timer

To defend against challenging physical and emotional demands, we often resort to protective posturing, such as rounding the shoulders and closing the chest. Supported Bridge Pose shows us gentle ways to open the chest and heart, the source of compassion and love. As you lie quietly over the bolsters, feel the soothing effects of placing your head lower than the rest of your body.

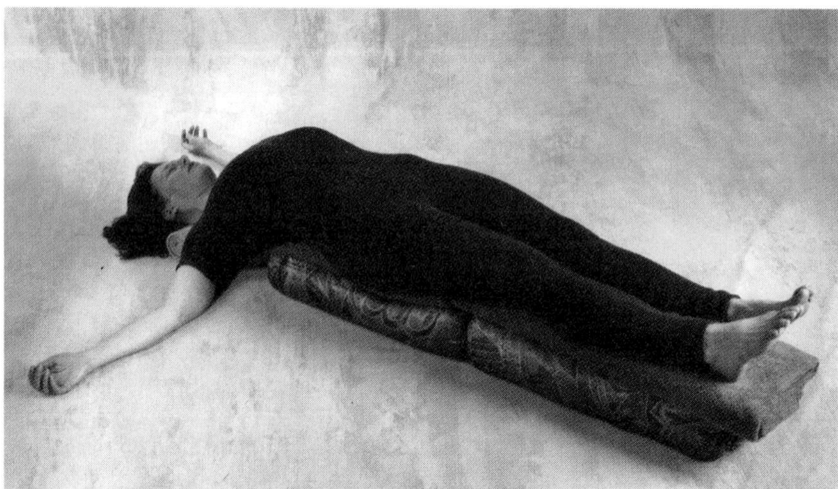

FIGURE 14.8
Supported Bridge Pose

Setting Up. See page 39 for a full discussion of setting up this pose.

Being There. Begin by making sure that you are comfortable. As you settle into the pose, turn your upper thighs inward, so it feels like the thigh bones drop toward the bolsters. Imagine that the hip bones also roll inward, so your belly feels like it is stretching toward the legs. When you do this, the belly, uterus, and ovaries drop down in the pelvic cavity.

Gently bring your attention to your breathing. Feel the lateral movement of your lungs and ribs with each inhalation and exhalation. To enhance your relaxation, let your eyeballs turn downward. Rest, poised between the energy of thought drawing inward and the energy of the body opening and expanding.

Coming Back. Practice Supported Bridge Pose as long as you are comfortable, up to 15 minutes. To come out, remove the eyebag and slide off the bolsters in the direction of your head. Rest your lower legs on the bolster, with your back on the floor. Stay for a few minutes, and then roll to one side. Press down with your hands and sit up slowly.

Benefits. In preliminary research, Supported Bridge Pose has been found to reduce blood levels of norepinephrine, a key hormone in the regulation of blood pressure.[2] Supported Bridge Pose is, therefore, positive for menopausal women, because elevated blood pressure often occurs when the protective effect of estrogen on blood pressure is withdrawn after menopause.

The action of dropping the belly, uterus, and ovaries in the pelvic cavity helps to balance hormonal secretions, thus moderating the hormonal swings of menopause.

In addition, Supported Bridge Pose is a mild inverted pose. It helps to drain fluid from the legs after long periods of standing, thus reducing fatigue.

Cautions

- If you get pregnant during perimenopause, do not practice this pose after the first three months.
- See page 40 for more advice on this inverted pose.

Supported Child's Pose

Because perimenopause often happens at a time of life when a woman is faced with many emotional demands, there will be times when you just want to climb in bed and pull the covers over your head. This is probably not possible most days (although I do recommend an occasional

Prop

- bolster

Optional Props

- 1 or more single-fold blankets
- 2 towels
- sandbag
- long-roll blanket
- extra blanket for warmth
- clock or timer

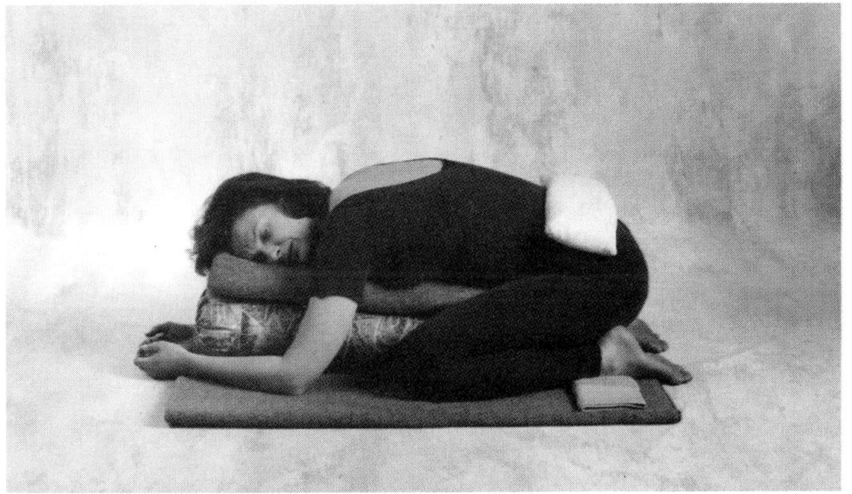

FIGURE 14.9
Supported Child's Pose

"pajama day"; see chapter 18). Try Supported Child's Pose instead. It offers the opportunity to take a rest in the middle of what feels like chaos.

Setting Up. See page 58 for details on setting up this pose.

Being There. Take several slow breaths. As you do, allow yourself to drop down and receive the support of the bolster. Let your belly relax. The counter-pressure of the bolster on the belly—as well as the sandbag on your lower back—may feel good if you have menstrual cramps. Continue to breathe and let your shoulders move away from the ears. Let the responsibilities of life roll off your back for the next few minutes as you rest in the safety of this egg shape. Trust your body to settle completely into the harmony of here and now—with no stress, no hot flashes, no insomnia—just the present moment.

Coming Back. Practice Supported Child's Pose for 1 to 3 minutes. Be sure that you spend an equal time with your head turned in each direction. Open your eyes, and place your palms on the floor, under your shoulders. Press your hands into the floor, inhale, and sit up slowly onto your heels. Rest for a moment. Come to a kneeling position, and immediately bring one leg forward, placing your foot on the floor. Press your hands on the forward thigh, and inhale deeply as you come to a standing position. Coming out of the pose in this way prevents discomfort in the knees.

Benefits. Supported Child's Pose creates a counterpressure on the abdomen and gently stretches the lower back. These actions relieve muscular tension during the irregular menstrual periods of perimenopause.

Caution

- See page 59 for advice on this pose.

All of the troubles of life come upon us because we refuse to sit quietly for a while each day in our rooms.
—BLAISE PASCAL

Basic Relaxation Pose with Sandbag and Bolster

Nothing is more important for the woman experiencing the transitions of menopause than the regular practice of relaxation. Not only does it soothe the physical symptoms, but it also mitigates emotional strain. The human body, regardless of its stage of development, functions more fully when stress is removed. Choosing to practice Basic Relaxation Pose each day sends a strong message to your unconscious that you deserve to live fully, calmly, and in physical and emotional harmony. As you practice, you experience that each moment of life is a transition.

Props

- standard-fold blanket
- sandbag
- bolster

Optional Props

- eyebag
- blanket or pillow to prop heels
- extra blanket for warmth
- clock or timer

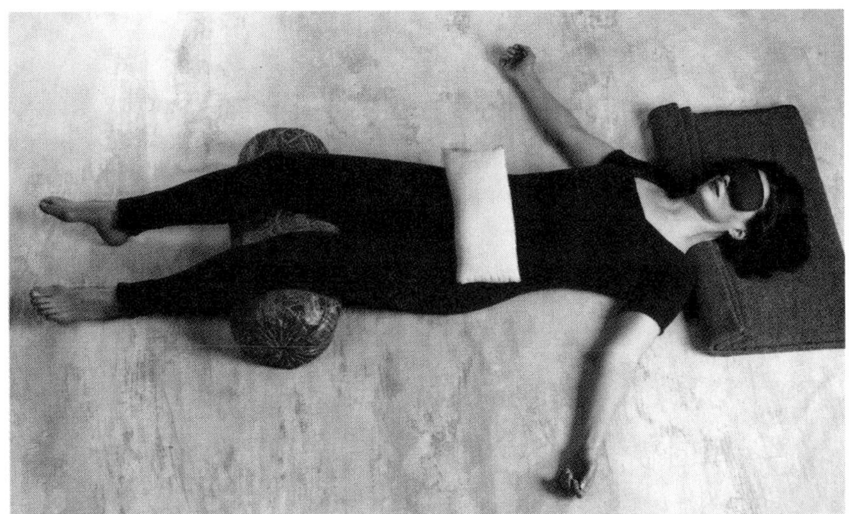

FIGURE 14.10
Basic Relaxation Pose with Sandbag and Bolster

Setting Up. See page 25 for basic instructions. In this variation, place a bolster under your knees before you lie down and a sandbag on your abdomen, over the navel area, once you are down.

Being There. As you rest, your arms and legs will feel longer and longer, as well as heavier. Feel the large muscles of the legs, buttocks, and trunk drop away from the bones. Now feel the smaller muscles of your arms, neck, and head, as they seem to move away from the bones. Let the bones themselves feel heavy and the skin loose, all over your body.

Accept the weight of the sandbag. As you do, it will feel lighter and lighter. When it does, this is a signal that you are ready to begin the Centering Breath. (See pages 24 and 26 for guidance in this breathing awareness technique.) Practice the Centering Breath for up to 10 rounds. Be sure to leave some time for normal breathing before coming out of the pose.

Coming Back. Practice Basic Relaxation Pose with Sandbag and Bolster for 7 to 20 minutes. To come out of the pose, slowly bend one knee and roll onto your side. Let the eyebag and sandbag fall off by themselves. Gradually open your eyes. Rest in this position for a few breaths. To sit up, press the floor with the elbow of your lower arm and the palm of the hand of your upper arm. Take a few breaths before standing up and resuming your normal activities.

Benefits. Basic Relaxation Pose with Sandbag and Bolster lowers blood pressure and heart rate, releases muscular tension, reduces fatigue, improves sleep, enhances immune response, and helps to manage chronic pain.

Cautions

- If you are having any amount of menstrual bleeding, do not practice with the sandbag over your belly.
- If you get pregnant during perimenopause, practice the Basic Relaxation Pose, described on page 25, during the first three months. After that, I recommend Side-Lying Relaxation Pose (see chapter 13).

PRACTICE SUMMARY

Here is a summary of the Opening to Menopause series, along with some suggestions on using poses from the series in shorter practice sessions.

60 to 100 Minutes

POSE	TIME
Wall Hang	1 minute
Hanging Dog Pose	1 to 2 minutes
Mountain Brook Pose	5 to 15 minutes
Supported Bound-Angle Pose	15 to 30 minutes
Elevated Legs-Up-the-Wall Pose	15 minutes
Supported Bridge Pose	15 minutes
Supported Child's Pose	1 to 2 minutes
Basic Relaxation Pose with Sandbag and Bolster	7 to 20 minutes

15 Minutes

POSE	TIME
Supported Bound-Angle Pose	15 minutes

20 Minutes

POSE	TIME
Supported Bridge Pose	5 minutes
Basic Relaxation Pose with Sandbag and Bolster	15 minutes

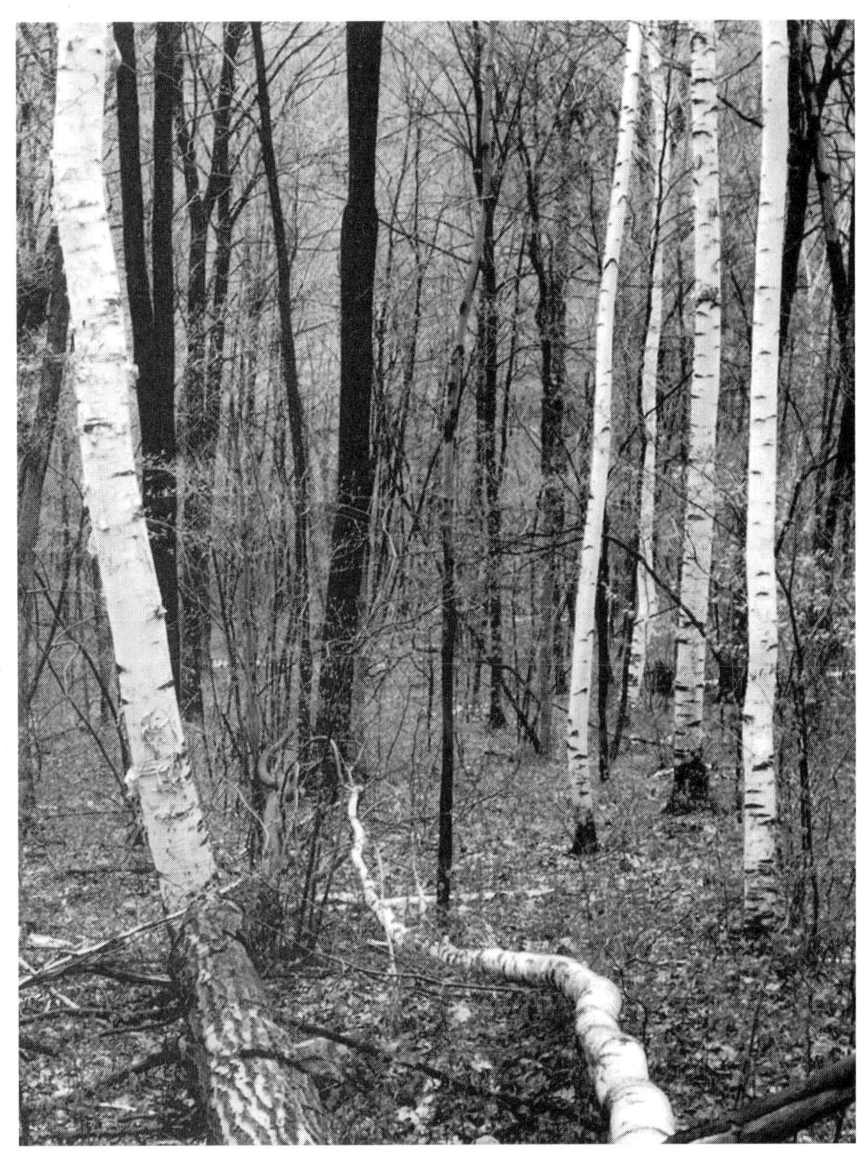

PART FOUR: LIVING YOUR YOGA

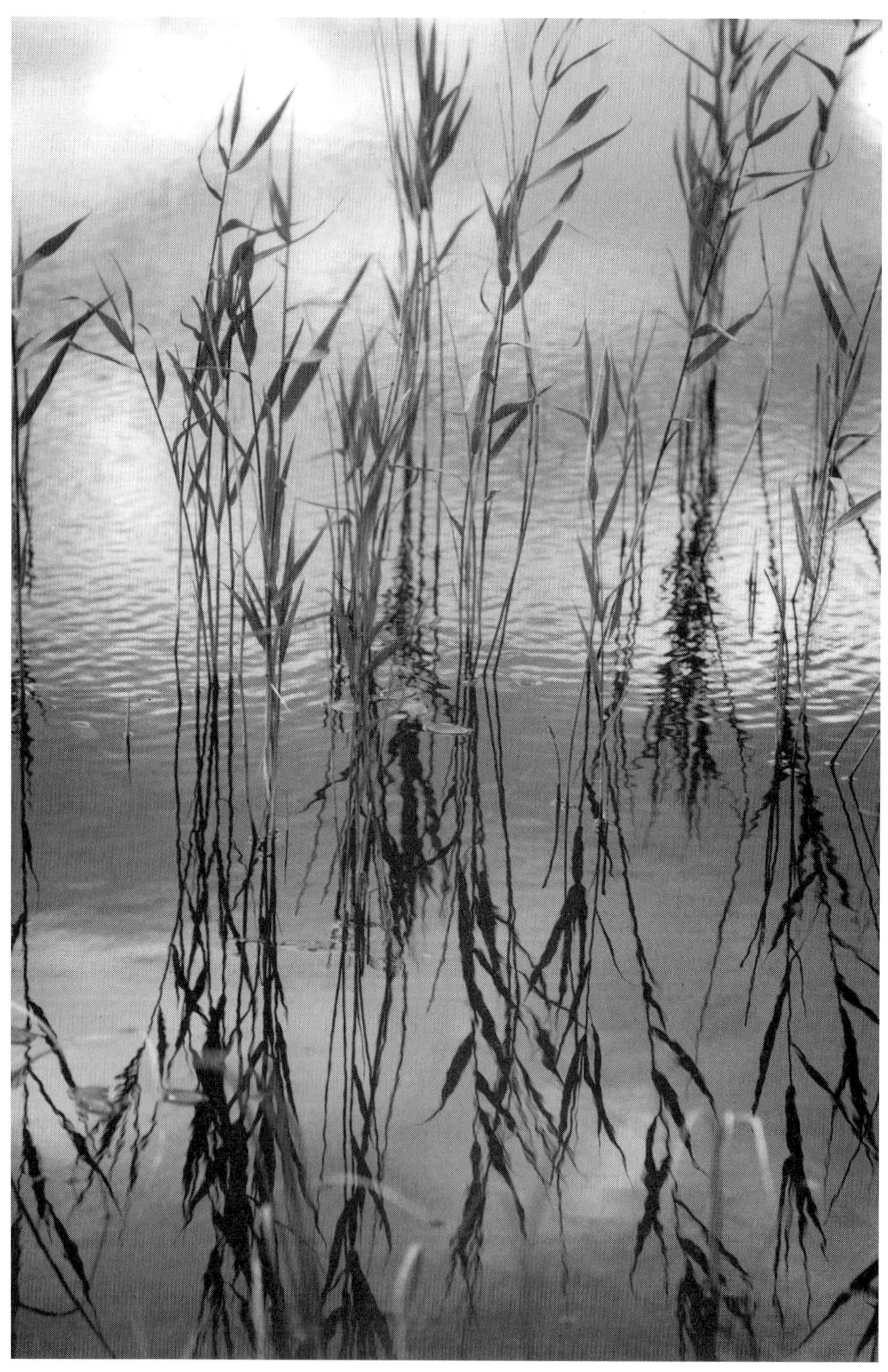

CHAPTER FIFTEEN

THE SILENT TEACHER

Watching the Breath

OUR PHYSICAL and mental states are reflected in the breath. In fact, there is no more reliable measurement of stress than the rate, depth, and quality of the breath. Under stressful conditions, the breath is shallow, rapid, and jagged. To change these qualities and therefore relieve stress, all you need to do is become aware of your breath. The simple act of bringing your attention to your breath changes it.

This chapter consists of a practice I call Living Your Yoga, a name I have given to numerous workshops I've taught since 1988. (And I wrote two books about these practices, entitled *Living Your Yoga and A Year of Living Your Yoga.*) In these workshops, we focus on bringing the principles of yoga practice into daily life. Here we explore ways to integrate breathing awareness into daily activities.

This practice further demonstrates the interconnection of mind and body. It can be said that the awareness developed through breathing practices is the beginning of meditation; some would say that it is meditation. This practice will bring you into the present, a moment when all of you—body, breath, and mind—can live your yoga.

Living Your Yoga

Body and soul are not two substances but one. They are man becoming aware of himself in two different ways.
—C.F. von Weizsacker

Throughout the book, we have practiced the Centering Breath while in the restorative poses. Here we focus on a practice to be done in the midst of your daily activities. Whenever you can, stop briefly and bring your attention to your breath. Claiming these few moments is important. When you are aware of your breath you are more present and have a more open perspective about the task at hand. What better tool can we bring to any task than awareness?

There are three ways to practice breathing awareness during your daily activities. First, notice your breath, nothing more. If you are sitting quietly, notice how little breath is required. If you are tense, the simple act of bringing your attention to your breath can be the first step in releasing your jaw and shoulders. If you are running, notice how the rapid and even breath fuels your body. If you are tired, this moment of attention could help you center and refresh yourself.

Second, you can use your breath to change your response to a situation. If you notice that you are holding your breath or breathing very rapidly, particularly in challenging situations, take slow, gentle breaths to calm down.

Third, observe your breath and let its rhythm guide you. For example, I often suggest to runners that they observe the rhythm of the breath as they begin running and then pace themselves at a speed compatible with that rhythm.

Your practice could be something you do regularly, like taking a few moments to breathe and enjoy the silence before getting out of bed in the morning. At other times, your practice may be in response to a particular situation, like pausing to breathe before speaking with someone you are annoyed with. Some suggestions about when to practice breathing awareness are given below. I have divided these suggestions into two categories: planned practice and response practice. As always, feel free to come up with ideas of your own.

Planned Practice

Bring your attention to your breath:

- before getting out of bed in the morning.
- just before you begin a meal.
- before picking up the receiver to make a telephone call.
- before you leave your house for work.
- before getting in your car.

- as you enter your workplace.
- when you come home.
- as you push around the grocery cart.
- before turning on television.
- when you pick up your child.
- when you sit down to help your child study.
- just before you go to sleep.

Response Practice

Bring your attention to your breath:

- during an intense conversation.
- during your child's temper tantrum.
- while waiting at a stop light.
- when someone cuts you off in traffic.
- whenever you think of someone you do not like.
- whenever you think you have too much to do in too little time.

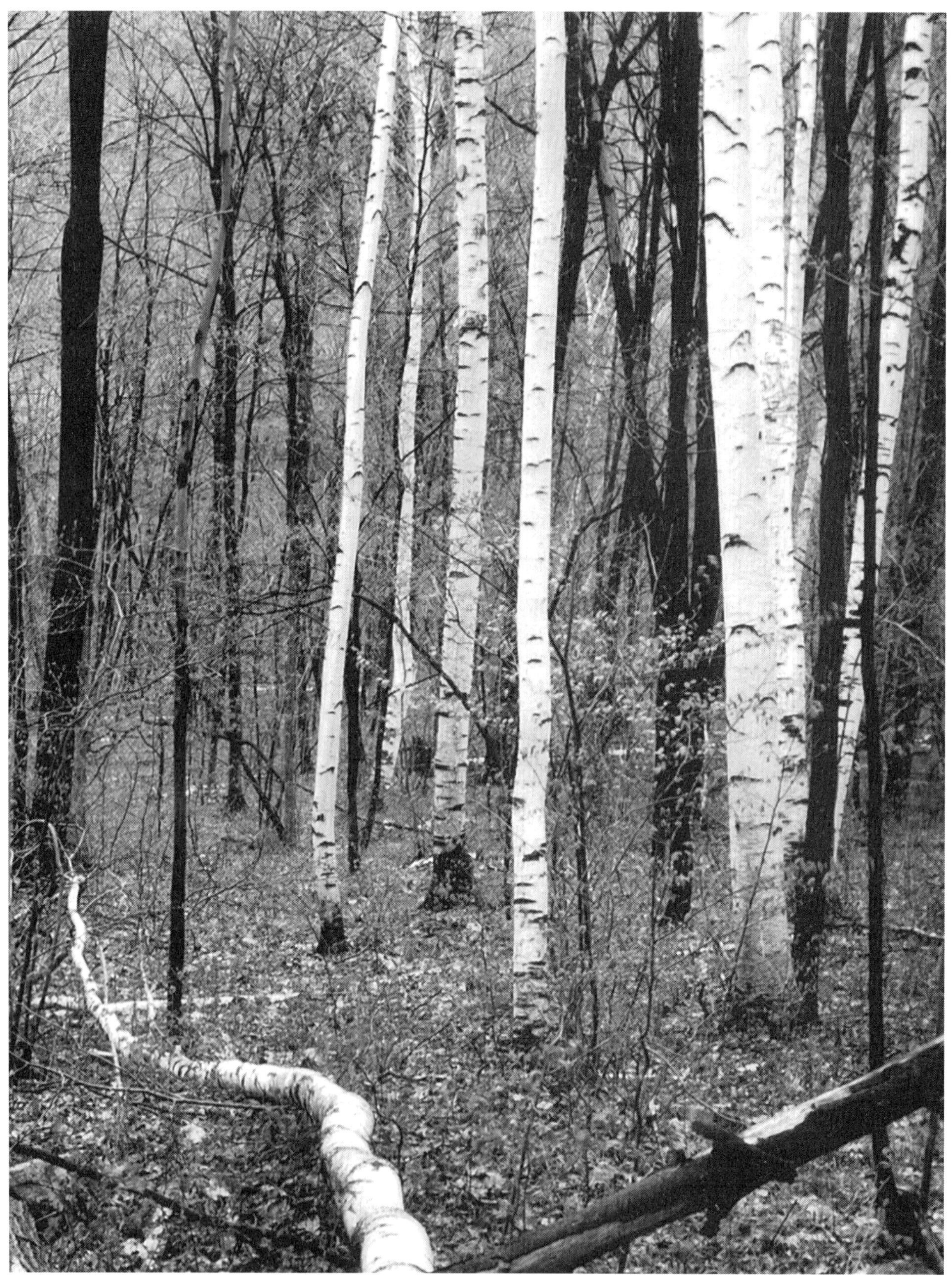

CHAPTER SIXTEEN

THE BACKBONE

Strength Through Curves

ONE OF THE most interesting structures in nature is the human spinal column. When the spine is well positioned, the unremitting force of gravity flows easily through it. If the spinal curves are habitually disturbed, gravity becomes the enemy. As a result, tension builds up around the spinal column, as the body attempts to hold itself upright by overusing muscles and ligaments. Since these structures were not intended exclusively for this use, the soft tissues of the back tire. This can lead to muscle spasms or generalized fatigue. One of the best ways to reduce stress is to stand so that the natural curves of the spine are maintained. In this chapter, we practice ways to do just that.

Commonly known as the backbone, the spinal column consists of thirty-two bones called vertebrae. They are arranged in a series of four gentle curves: cervical (neck), thoracic (middle back), lumbar (lower back), and sacro-coccygeal (pelvis). In order to bear weight successfully, these curves should neither be increased nor decreased too much.

Most of the vertebrae are separated by intervertebral discs, which are pads of fibrocartilage. All are connected by ligaments, or bands of connective tissue, and muscles that enable us to twist and bend forward, backward, and sideways. In between the vertebrae are the exit points for the spinal nerves, which branch from the spinal cord itself. The spinal cord passes through the middle of the spinal column, ending at the level of the first lumbar vertebra.

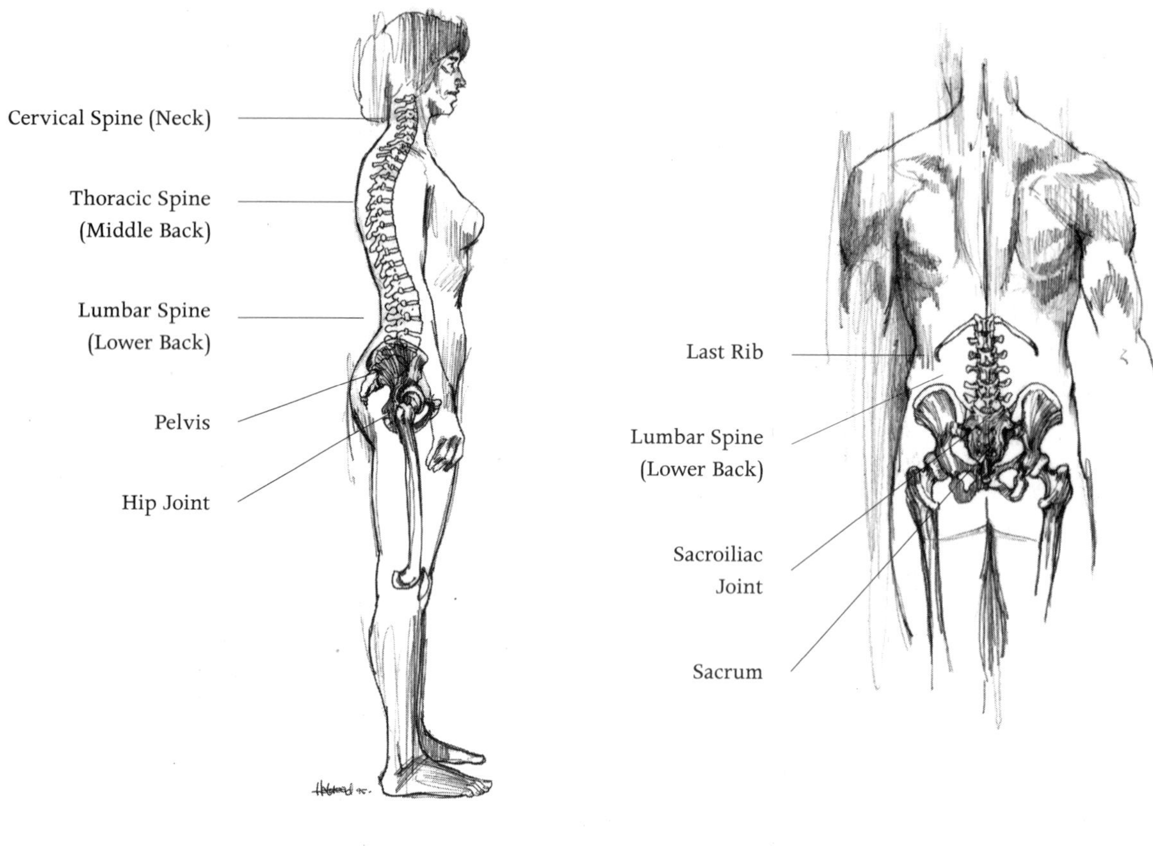

FIGURE 16.1
Vertebral Column, Side View

FIGURE 16.2
Pelvis, Back View

For some hands-on information about the spine, stand sideways near a full-length mirror. The spine begins at the base of the skull and ends at the tailbone. Begin by running your fingertips from the base of your skull gently down the back of your neck. Feel how your neck curves toward the front of your body. This is called the cervical spine, and it consists of seven vertebrae.

The next region of the spine is called the thoracic spine. Look in the mirror and notice how your upper back curves away from your body in exactly the opposite direction from your neck. There are twelve thoracic vertebrae, each with two ribs attached.

Below the thoracic region is the lumbar spine, or lower back. It extends from the last rib in the back to the top of the sacrum. The lumbar spine has five vertebrae and, like the cervical vertebrae at the top of the spine, curves inward. Place your fingers at the back of your waist and feel this gentle curve.

Let your fingers continue down the back until you locate the sacrum, a triangular-shaped bone that curves outward like the thoracic spine. Unique in composition, the sacrum consists of five vertebrae that fused together during the normal course of development. Below the sacrum are three small bones that make up the coccyx, or tailbone. They are inconsequential to most spinal movements. The only time most of us think about the tailbone is when we fall on it.

::: PRACTICE

Standing Well: Mountain Pose

In yoga, standing in the position of postural awareness is called Mountain Pose. When this pose is practiced well, the body is prepared for

Prop

- nonskid floor or mat

Optional

- mirror
- a friend

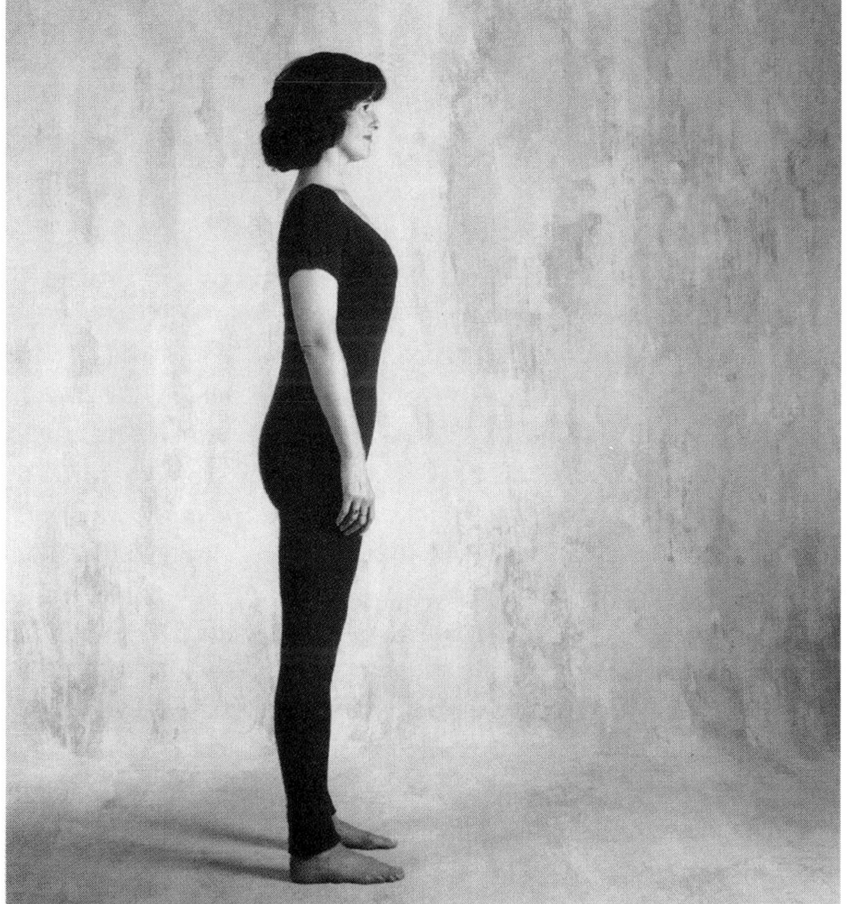

FIGURE 16.3
Mountain Pose

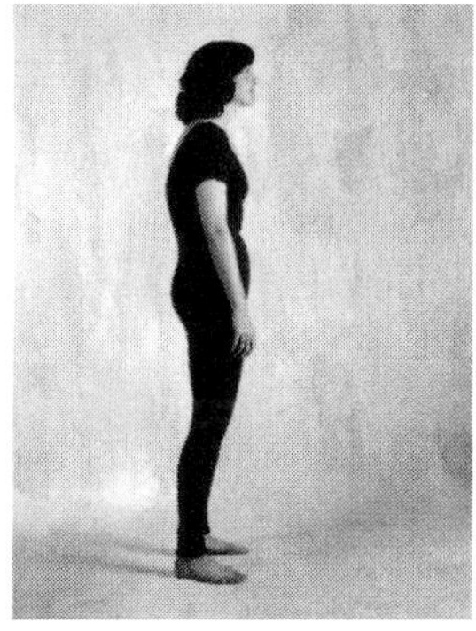

FIGURE 16.4
Mountain Pose, Incorrect

almost all daily movement: standing, sitting, walking, and running. Like the mountain poised between heaven and earth, this pose establishes a foundation through the legs and feet and encourages the lift of the spine.

Setting Up. Stand sideways near a full-length mirror so you can check your alignment. Alternatively, practice with a friend who can tell you how you are doing. If you find yourself without these props, practice anyway. The more you practice, the more you will develop an internal sense of your own alignment.

We begin with the foundation: your feet. Attention to the details of placing the feet is important. Stand with your feet hip-width apart. For most people, this is about 6 to 10 inches. The center line of the foot should point forward. If you are not sure what this means, look down and imagine that each foot is placed on a line drawn from a point between your second and third toes through the center of the front of your ankle and continuing to the center of your heel.

Standing with your feet parallel can help to maintain the normal spinal curves and a balanced position of the pelvis. Standing with the feet turned out causes the back of the pelvis to drop and flattens the lumbar curve. Standing with the feet turned in tilts the top of the pelvis forward, increases the lumbar curve, and stresses the inner knees.

After you have positioned your feet, place your hands on the rim of your pelvis. If you are not sure where this is, put your hands at the sides of your waist and slowly move them down until you feel a bony ridge. This is the rim of the pelvis.

With your hands on the pelvic rim, feel if the pelvis is in a balanced position. If you have pushed the pelvis backward, you flatten the lumbar curve, decrease the ability of the lumbar spine to bear weight successfully, and increase strain on the soft tissues in the area. To correct this misalignment, adjust the pelvis so that it sits exactly over the tops of the thighs. Correct alignment may feel strange at first, so check yourself in the mirror or ask your friend for feedback. Looking at you from the side, your friend should be able to draw an imaginary vertical line from your ear to your shoulder joint and down through the center of your hip, knee, and ankle. Once you have found a good position for the pelvis, let your arms drop to your sides.

The body is mortal. It is subject to death. Yet it is the resting place of the immortal, incorporeal Self.
—Chandogya Upanishad

Do not hyperextend your knees. Commonly called locking the knees, hyperextension is a position in which you hang backward on the internal knee ligaments. This habitual posture overstretches these ligaments and leads to instability in the knee joints. If you stand this way, bend your knees slightly to avoid pushing back. Check in the mirror to make sure that your lower legs are vertical.

Now bring your attention to your head and neck. If the body is aligned, usually the head follows. But take a moment to check it anyway. This is harder to do by yourself, so ask a friend for feedback. If you are practicing on your own, here are two ways you can check the position of your head and neck.

First, your eyes should be level with the horizon. If you are looking up or down, even slightly, your head is tipped, and your neck will not be in a neutral position. Remember, in its neutral position the cervical spine has a slight inward curve.

Man is not disturbed by things, but by his opinions about things.
—EPICTETUS

Second, place your fingers at the base of your skull to help you feel the position of the back of your skull in relationship to your neck. Is the skull moving down toward the neck? If you are not sure, exaggerate the movement. Notice how your chin juts forward and you feel increased tension in the muscles of the back of your neck. Bring your head back to the point where the skull lifts away from the neck and the chin is parallel to the floor. As you do this, feel the neck muscles soften.

Being There. Once you are in alignment, notice your physical sensations. Is your weight balanced evenly between your feet? Between the fronts and backs of your feet? Your legs should feel active, but not tight. Is there any tension in your shoulders? Drop them away from your ears, and allow your arms to feel long and relaxed at your sides.

Feel a lightness in your spinal column and the exhilaration from the upward movement of the spine. Allow your head to be balanced on your torso.

Feel minimum effort and maximum comfort in breathing. Breathe several long, smooth breaths and relax, still maintaining awareness of your alignment.

Benefits. Practice Mountain Pose several times a day. Standing well reduces strain on the joints, ligaments, and muscles, especially on those of the spinal column and lower extremities. It also aids respiration, digestion, and elimination. It gives you confidence and conveys a sense of poise and self-esteem.

Cautions

- Remove your socks for this pose.
- If you have low blood pressure, do not practice Mountain Pose for more than 2 minutes.

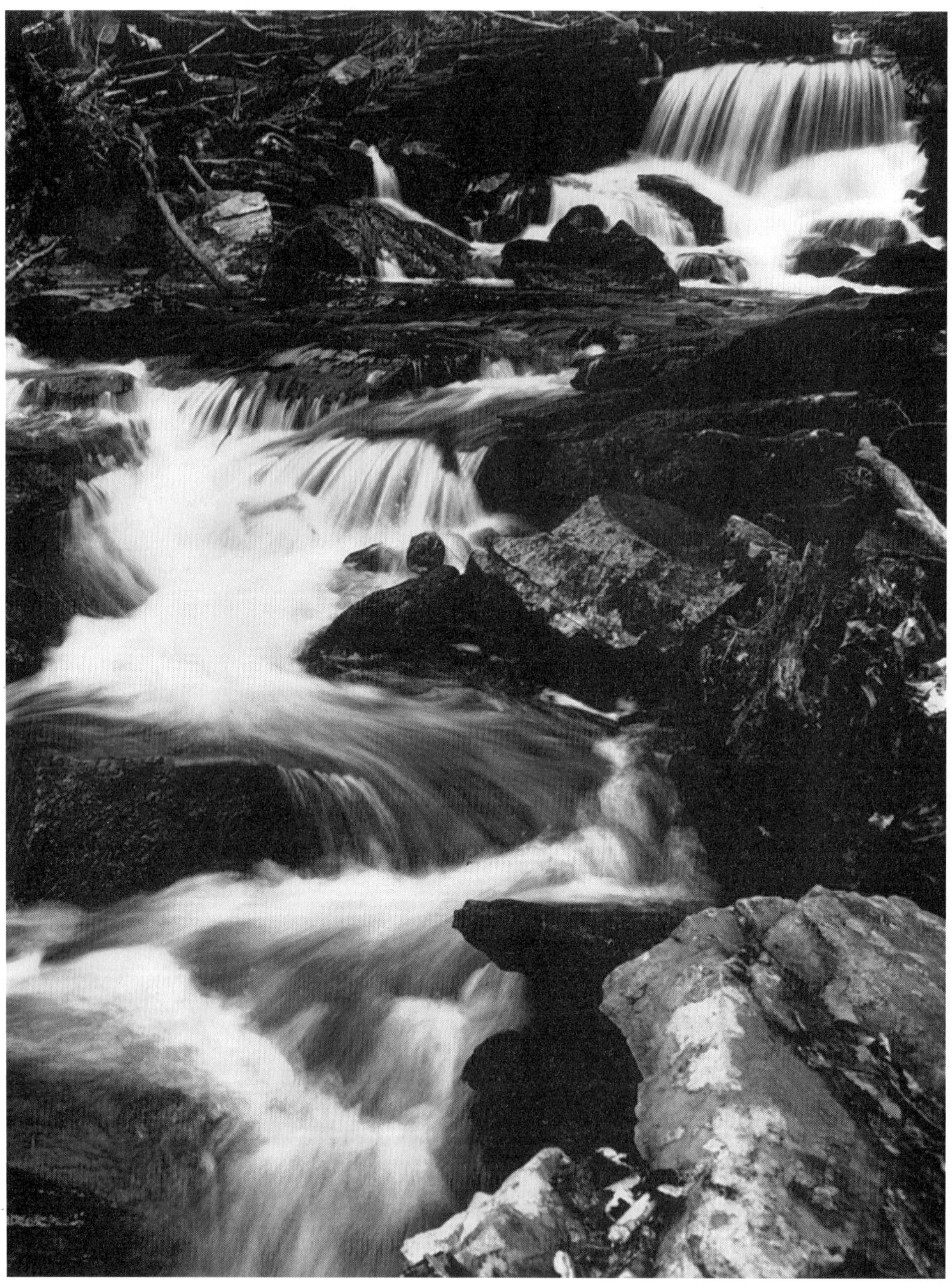

CHAPTER SEVENTEEN

SITTING PRETTY

Making Friends with a Chair

■ ■ ■

As we discussed in chapter 16, one of the best ways to reduce stress is to stand in a manner that maintains the natural curves of the spinal column. When the curves are at their optimum, there is maximum stability and minimum strain on the entire spine. Applying this principle to sitting is even more difficult than to standing because of that ever-variable invention, the chair.

Chairs comes in wood, metal, or plastic, with straight, curved, and slanted backs, and with or without armrests. Most are designed to accommodate the "average person," that is, someone five feet six in height. Is it any wonder that most of us do not feel comfortable in chairs or on the sofa? Traveling in cars, buses, trains, or airplanes is no exception. What do you do if you are not "average"? What if your feet do not reach the floor when you sit or your knees are up to your chin? What do you do if the armrests are too high? What if you have to sit for long periods of time?

In this chapter, we explore ways to sit that maintain the natural curves of the spinal column, no matter what surface you're sitting on. Remember, the cervical (neck), thoracic (midback), and lumbar (lower back) curves are interrelated. If one curve changes, the others follow suit. With this in mind, let's consider what can happen to posture when you are sitting.

To understand posture, one experience is worth a thousand words. If you are not already sitting, take this book with you to your favorite chair and sit down as you normally would. Spend a few moments getting comfortable. How are you sitting? You are probably not sitting solidly on your sitting bones (ischial tuberosities), but are rolled back onto your tailbone or your sacrum in a "slumped" position. Place your hand on your lumbar curve (lower back), located at the level of your waist. Feel how it flattens or reverses from its natural position. Notice how your chest has collapsed; feel how your head and neck jut forward.

How does it feel to sit this way? Not too good? You're right. Your vertebrae and discs are compressed, your muscles and ligaments are stressed, and your breathing capacity is reduced. In this position, you will tire more easily. When combining this posture with other factors—for example, the mental demands of your job—the seemingly routine activity of sitting becomes a most stressful event.

Sitting well is essential for maintaining a healthy spine. In this chapter, we practice Seated Mountain Pose. I encourage you to integrate this pose into your daily life of work, study, and leisure. Some practical suggestions at the end of the chapter can help you get started.

::: PRACTICE

Seated Mountain Pose

Props

- chair

Optional Props

- blocks or a stack of books
- double-fold blanket
- 1 or more towels
- 1 or more pillows

Seated Mountain Pose applies the principles of alignment and awareness that you practiced in Mountain Pose (see chapter 16) to a seated position. Practice this pose as part of your restorative routine. You can begin the Relax and Renew practice session, presented in chapter 5, with a few minutes of Seated Mountain Pose. It's a good way to develop proper sitting habits and a creative transition from your normal daily activities into your practice time.

Setting Up. Stand in Mountain Pose, close to your chair. Bring one foot back slightly, if possible. Using the strength of your legs, bend your knees and maintain the normal curves of your spine, as you gently lower your torso. Sit on the front half of your chair seat. Position your feet so they rest on the floor and are parallel. Make sure that your legs are comfortably apart.

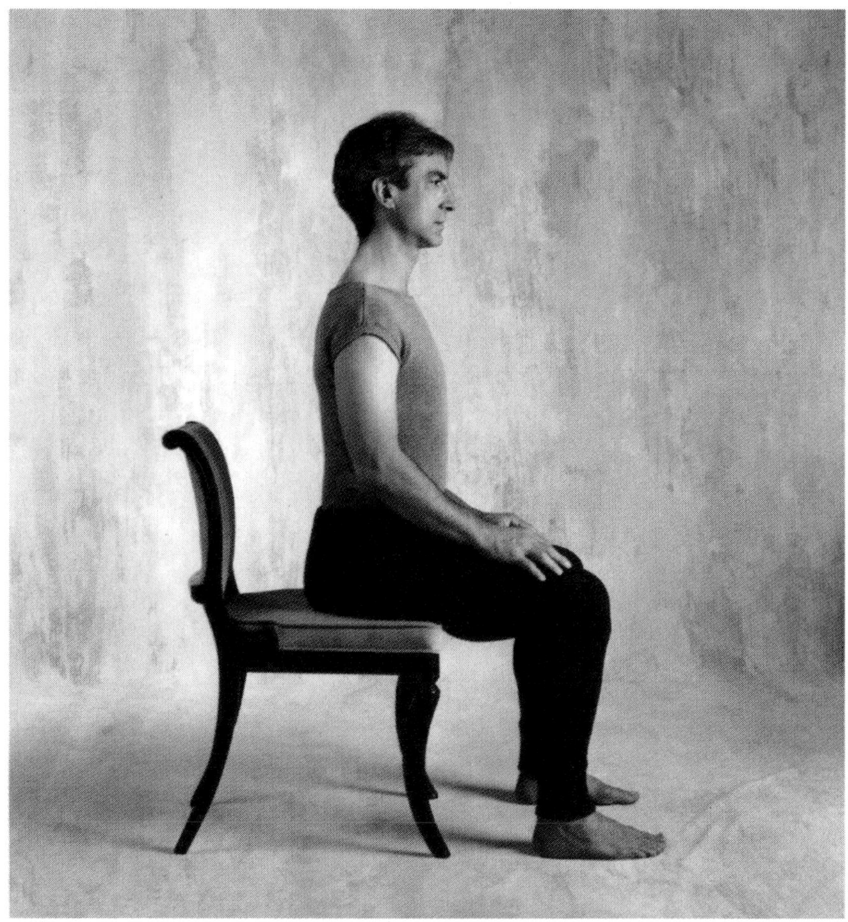

FIGURE 17.1 Seated Mountain Pose

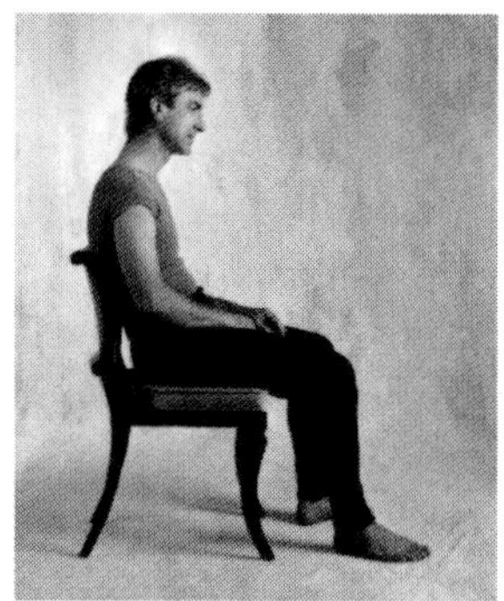

FIGURE 17.2
Seated Mountain Pose, Incorrect

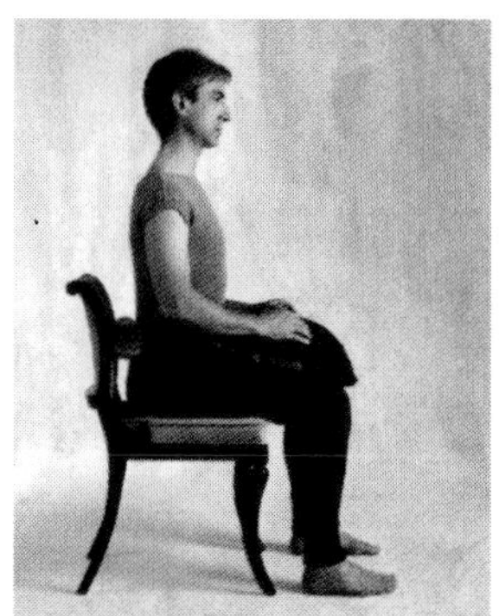

FIGURE 17.3
Seated Mountain Pose, Variation

If your situation does not allow you to sit forward in the chair, you may sit back, but make sure your knees are comfortably apart and your feet are either flat on the floor or resting on a support. If the feet dangle, it is impossible to relax. The support should be high enough so your thigh bones are parallel to the floor. A stack of books works well. If you are sitting back in the chair, you can also place a rolled towel at your lower back to maintain your lumbar curve and another behind your neck to maintain the cervical curve. Experiment with the thickness of the rolls, so the props are just right for you.

Place your forearms on the armrests, so that your shoulders relax away from your ears. If the chair has no armrests or if they are too high for you, let your hands rest comfortably in your lap. If this feels uncomfortable, place one or more pillows on your lap, and rest your hands and forearms on that. Use enough support so your shoulders, head, and neck are free.

Your worst enemy cannot harm you as much as your thoughts unguarded.
—SHAKYAMUNI BUDDHA

Being There. Have you ever watched an 8-to-10-month-old baby sit? Remember how effortlessly she held her head, neck, and spine? Let your body respond to this image as you practice Seated Mountain Pose.

Bring your attention to your spinal column, which runs from the base of the head to the tip of the tailbone. Begin at the lumbar area. It should curve gently inward, just as when you stand correctly. Purposely round your lower back and experience how your entire spinal column follows the lumbar collapse. Now bring your lower back into proper alignment, and feel how your whole spine responds by lifting upward. This does not mean you should force or exaggerate the position of the lumbar spine. It is just as unhealthy to arch too much as it is to arch too little.

If the chair you are using makes it impossible to keep the lumbar curve in its natural alignment, place a folded towel under your sitting bones to tip your pelvis forward. Adjust the support so that your pelvis is slightly higher than your thighs. (Kneeling-style chairs—with slanted seats and separate pads on which to rest the knees—are designed to do exactly this.)

Once you are sitting with a normal lumbar curve, allow your thoracic curve to round outward. This adjustment is a moderate one. Feel the freedom that comes to your ribs and to your breathing. Feel your cervical spine curving gently inward and the sense of ease that comes to the neck and throat.

Take a few moments to assess your overall comfort level. You will know when you are sitting well because you will feel the results: spine effortlessly long, chest lifting, ribs hanging from the shoulders, and head and neck poised easily over the body. Take several deep breaths. The breath should come easily. You should feel pleasantly relaxed.

Coming Back. You can practice Seated Mountain Pose for several minutes. To come out of the chair, move to the edge of the seat and place one foot slightly under it. Do not lead with your chin, but try to maintain the normal curves of the spine as you stand up.

Benefits. Seated Mountain Pose helps you breathe more freely and digest more easily. It increases mental alertness.

Caution

- Do not let the pose become rigid. If you feel any pain or discomfort, come out of the pose.

Sitting Well All Day Long

Here are a few practical suggestions to help you take Seated Mountain Pose into your daily life.

- Have a few props to use at your place of work or study.
- If you sit for long periods of time—at work, to study, watching television, or listening to music—make sure you take breaks at frequent intervals and take a short walk, even if it is around the room.
- When working at a desk or table, avoid the temptation to slouch. Elevate your papers or book so you do not have to drop your head to read.
- Bring your rolled towel to an evening at the movies. Place it at your lumbar spine to help maintain its natural curve.
- Keep a spare rolled towel in your car. Use it to support your lumbar curve, no matter how short the trip.
- If you are traveling by train or airplane, bring along a rolled towel to support your lumbar curve. If you left it at home, ask an attendant for a blanket to use.
- If your sport of choice is rowing, bicycling, or another seated one, and it is obviously not possible to use props, try to apply the principles of healthful spinal alignment. You are probably rounding the thoracic curve too much, so take frequent stretch breaks.
- Use Seated Mountain Pose as a meditation position: breathe, center, be quiet, and relax.

Some remedies are worse than the disease.
—Publilius Syrus

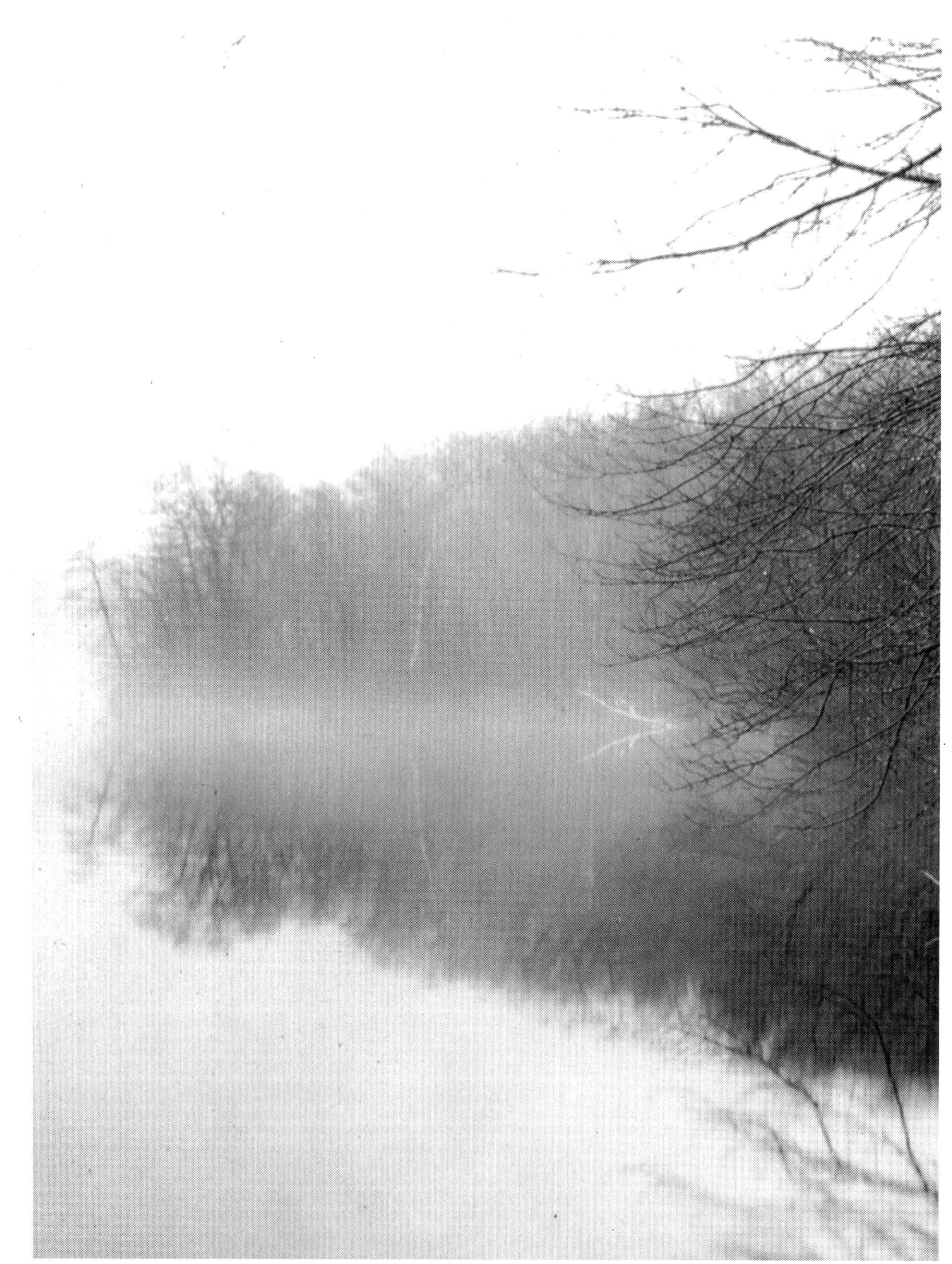

CHAPTER EIGHTEEN

STRESS-PROOF YOUR LIFE

Mindful Ways to Relax

IN A STUDY conducted at the department of psychiatry at the State University of New York at Stony Brook, one hundred volunteers were asked to compile a list of their daily positive and negative experiences. When researchers compared this information with antibody activity in volunteers' saliva (which indicates immune function), they discovered that stress from a negative event affects the immune system on the day it happens; a positive one can boost the system for two days or more.[1]

My prescription for reducing stress in your life: decide here and now that you are your own first priority. We each have the same twenty-four hours in a day and can make choices about how to live them. There are many simple, low- or no-cost things that you can do to reduce stress, and I have given you a few suggestions. Some are gentle reminders to relax that you can do often, even daily; others require some planning. They are all intended to help you slow down, take care of yourself, and relax and renew. Your reward will be twofold: you'll feel good in the moment and for the next few days.

Gentle Reminders

I am beginning to learn that it is the sweet, simple things of life which are the real ones after all.
—LAURA INGALLS WILDER

Choose something you feel you can actually do over the next several days. Write your choice on a note and stick it on a mirror, the refrigerator, the dashboard of your car, or in another place where you will be sure to see it. For example, "I will drive within the speed limit." You may want to post a reminder in more than one place. After several days, take some time to reflect on what you have noticed since you began this practice. You may decide to continue with it as it is, or to modify it, or to move on to a new one. Use the suggestions here, or make some of your own.

- Ask for help when you need it.
- Drive within the speed limit.
- Be willing to say, "I don't know."
- In a stressful situation, ask yourself this question, "What is the most important thing right now?"
- Position the interior rearview mirror in your car so you have to stretch a little to look in it. This will remind you to lengthen your spine and not collapse when driving. Write on your posted note: "Breathe."
- When you feel yourself pushing to complete a self-imposed task, ask yourself this question, "Will this matter in a year?"
- Take several long, slow breaths at every stop light.
- Notice how often you say "Hurry up!" to yourself or someone else, especially a child.
- Drive in the slow lane; avoid the fast lane, especially if you are in a hurry.
- Remember, the only people who are finished with everything are dead.

Make a Plan to Relax

Stress-proof your life by making plans to relax. If you are unable to take a holiday or a long break, here are a few things you can do to reduce stress, whether for a few minutes or a few hours.

- Practice Basic Relaxation Pose for 5 minutes several days a week.
- Eat breakfast every day.
- Take a nap each Saturday.
- Take a walk in the park in the middle of the week. Do not wear your watch.
- Buy flowers for yourself once a week.

- Leave for your appointment 10 minutes earlier than usual and enjoy the trip.
- Take a walk with a young child. Walk at his pace. Stop whenever he wants to stop, for as long as he wants. Notice if you feel impatient. Let him teach you how to slow down.
- Do not take a working vacation, and be sure to use your vacation time in the year you have accrued it.
- Agree to meet someone between two times, for example, between 1:00 and 1:30, instead of at an exact time. Give yourself some leeway.
- Read a book not related to your work and not about self-improvement or any project.
- Take your lunch break away from your desk. There is always more to be done; don't sacrifice nourishing yourself.
- Plan a "pajama day," when you stay home in your pajamas and do whatever you want. You could read, soak in the tub, or listen to music. Let your answering machine take your telephone calls.
- Write a letter to someone you miss. Use special paper and pen. Take your time.
- Lie on the couch for several minutes. Do not listen to music, read, talk on the phone, or sleep. Just be there.
- Take a 5-minute stretch break at work. Remember to breathe.
- Decide on one task that you would like to accomplish by a certain date. Write it in your datebook. Make a realistic plan of how to meet your deadline, and then stop nagging yourself about it.

Silence is another form of sound.
—Jane Hollister Wheelwright

APPENDIX

RESOURCES

WHETHER YOU ARE LOOKING for the camaraderie of a yoga class or need a yoga bolster, these resources will help you relax and renew.

Relax and Renew Seminars
with Judith Lasater, Ph.D., P.T.

These seminars are open to individuals, yoga teachers, and health care professionals. For more information, visit www.judithlasater.com and www.restorativeyogateachers.com.

Where to Find Yoga Teacher

If you want to study with a yoga teacher either privately or in a class setting, choose wisely. A competent teacher is professional, compassionate, knowledgeable, and maintains a personal yoga practice. All of the teachers listed in the directory on www.restorativeyogateachers.com have completed training with Judith Hanson Lasater.

Books

Back Care Basics
Mary Pullig Schatz, M.D.
Berkeley, CA: Rodmell Press, 1992
Learn practical ways to heal your back and neck, restructure your body, and manage stress with a doctor's gentle yoga program for back and neck pain relief. 200 photos and illustrations. Softcover, 248 pages.

Light on Pranayama
B.K.S. Iyengar
New York: Crossroad, 1981
A clear, detailed account of the yogic art of breathing, together with a comprehensive background of yoga philosophy. Softcover, 294 pages.

Yoga: A Gem for Women
Geeta S. Iyengar
Spokane, WA: Timeless Books, 1987
A comprehensive approach to hatha yoga, including special instructions for menstruation and pregnancy. 215 photographs. Softcover, 308 pages.

Yoga for Pregnancy
Judith Hanson Lasater, Ph.D., P.T.
Berkeley, CA: Rodmell Press, 2003
Yoga poses and breathing practices to help the mother to stay flexible and healthy throughout pregnancy, remain present during the challenges of labor and delivery, and care for herself during the postpartum period. Special section: "Mantras for Mom and Baby," where the mother can explore heart-centered practices, one for each month during pregnancy and baby's first year. 13 photographs. Softcover, 64 pages.

Website

North American Menopause Society
www.menopause.org
A free online resource for midlife women.

Props

Hugger-Mugger Yoga Products
(800) 473-4888
www.huggermugger.com

RECOMMENDED READING

Here is a list of wonderful books that have my heartfelt recommendation. Some books discuss practical approaches to help you care for your body, such as exercise and nutrition; others guide you in time-honored practices, such as meditation and prayer. Still others explore the tender subjects of disease, pain, and illness in ways that will leave you feeling comforted. Spend some time with those that speak to your needs. Each book will, in its own way, nurture you—body and soul.

Body/Mind

Borysenko, Joan. *Minding the Body, Mending the Mind.* New York: Warner Books, 1990.

Chopra, Deepak, M.D. *Ageless Body, Timeless Mind.* New York: Harmony Books, 1993.

———. *Creating Health.* Boston: Houghton Mifflin, 1991a.

———. *Perfect Health.* New York: Harmony Books, 1991b.

———. *Quantum Healing.* New York: Bantam Books, 1989.

Dossey, Larry, M.D. *Healing Words.* San Francisco: HarperSanFrancisco, 1993.

Kabat-Zinn, Jon. *Full Catastrophe Living.* New York: Doubleday/Dell, 1990.

Laskow, Leonard, M.D. *Healing with Love.* San Francisco: HarperSanFrancisco, 1992.

Spiegel, David, M.D. *Living Beyond Limits.* New York: Times Books, 1993.

Health/General

Connor, Sonja L., and William E. Connor, M.D. *The New American Diet.* New York: Simon and Schuster, 1991.

Ornish, Dean, M.D. *Dr. Dean Ornish's Program for Reversing Heart Disease.* New York: Random House, 1990.

———. *Eat More, Weigh Less.* New York: HarperCollins, 1993.

———. *Stress, Diet, and Your Heart.* Boston: Houghton Mifflin, 1984.

Rapoport, Alan M., M.D., and Fred D. Sheftell, M.D. *Headache Relief.* New York: Simon and Schuster, 1990.

Health/Women

Greenwood, Sadja, M.D. *Menopause, Naturally.* Rev. ed. San Francisco: Volcano Press, 1993.

Noble, Elizabeth. *Essential Exercises for the Childbearing Year.* 3d ed. Boston: Houghton Mifflin, 1988.

Inspiration

Haidt, Jonathan. *The Happiness Hypothesis.* New York: Basic Books, 2006.

Kornfield, Jack. *Buddha's Little Instruction Book.* New York: Bantam Books, 1994.

Lara, Adair. *Slowing Down in a Speeded-Up World.* Emeryville, CA: Conari Press, 1994.

Peisner, Paula. *Finding Time.* Napierville, Ill.: Sourcebooks Trade, 1992.

Meditation

Beck, Charlotte Joko. *Everyday Zen.* Edited by Steve Smith. San Francisco: Harper and Row, 1989.

Beck, Charlotte Joko, with Steve Smith. *Nothing Special.* San Francisco: HarperSanFrancisco, 1993.

Kabat-Zinn, Jon. *Wherever You Go, There You Are.* New York: Hyperion, 1994.

Kornfield, Jack. *A Path with Heart.* New York: Bantam Books, 1993.

Moore, Thomas. *Care of the Soul.* New York: HarperCollins, 1992.

Relaxation

Benson, Herbert, M.D. *The Relaxation Response.* New York: William Morrow and Company, 1975.

Benson, Herbert, M.D., Eileen M. Stuart, and the Staff of the Mind/Body Institute of New England Deaconess Hospital and Harvard Medical School. *The Wellness Book.* New York: Carol Publishing Group, 1992.

Davis, Martha, Elizabeth Robbins Eshelman, and Matthew McKay. *The Relaxation and Stress Reduction Workbook.* Oakland, CA: New Harbinger Publications, 1990.

Jacobson, Edmund, M.D. *You Must Relax.* 5th ed. New York: McGraw Hill, 1978.

Sapolsky, Robert M. *Why Zebras Don't Get Ulcers.* New York: W. H. Freeman and Company, 1993.

Yoga Philosophy

Mishra, Rammurti, M.D. *The Textbook of Yoga Psychology.* Edited by Ann Adman. New York: Julian Press, 1963.

Prabhavananda, Swami, and Christopher Isherwood. *How to Know God.* New York: New American Library, 1953.

NOTES

Chapter 1

1. Edmund Jacobson, M.D., *You Must Relax* (New York: McGraw-Hill, 1934).
2. Herbert Benson, M.D., Eileen M. Stuart, and the staff of the Mind/Body Institute of New England Deaconess Hospital and Harvard Medical School, *The Wellness Book* (New York: Carol Publishing, 1992), 36.
3. David Spiegel, M.D., *Living Beyond Limits* (New York: Times Books, 1993), 92–93.
4. For an enlightening discussion of body-mind medicine, see Deepak Chopra, M.D., *Quantum Healing* (New York: Bantam Books, 1989).
5. Dean Ornish, M.D., *Dr. Dean Ornish's Program for Reversing Heart Disease* (New York: Random House, 1990).
6. B.K.S Iyengar, *Light on Yoga* (New York: Schocken Books, 1979).
7. Roger Cole, personal communication with author, 3 August 1994.

Chapter 5

1. Samkhya-yogacharya Swami Hariharananda, *The Yoga Philosophy of Patanjali* (Albany, NY: State University of New York Press, 1983), 327.

Chapter 7

1. F. T. Dagi and J. F. Beary, "Low Back Pain," in *Rheumatology and Outpatient Disorders,* ed. J. F. Beary, 2d ed. (Boston: Little Brown, 1987), 97–103.
2. Laurie McGinley, "Acute Back Pain Calls for Mild Exercise, Painkillers, Not Surgery, Panel Reports," *Wall Street Journal,* 9 December 1994, sec. B, p. 3.
3. Ibid.

Chapter 8

1. J. N. Blau, M.D., *Overcoming Headaches and Migraines* (Stamford, CT: Longmeadow Press, 1993), 31.
2. N. Vijayan, M.D., "Head Band for Migraine Headache Relief," *Headache* 33, no. 1 (January 1993): 40–41.

Chapter 9

1. Roger Cole, Ph.D., personal communication with author, 3 August 1994.

Chapter 10

1. Bernard J. Colan, "Researchers Explore Therapeutic Effects of Yoga," *Advance,* 5 April 1993, 19.
2. Janet Bailey, "Anxious Breathing," *Glamour,* January 1995, 28.

Chapter 11

1. Dan A. Oren, M.D., et al., *How to Beat Jet Lag* (New York: Henry Holt and Company, 1993), 2–3.

Chapter 12

1. Madeline Drexler, "What Can You Do About Endometriosis?" *Self,* January 1995, 122–23, 139.
2. Boston Women's Health Collective, *The New Our Bodies, Ourselves* (New York: Simon and Schuster, 1992), 586.

Chapter 13

1. Stephanie Young, "Why You're So Tired," *Glamour,* January 1995, 44.

Chapter 14

1. In Gail Sheehy, *The Silent Passage,* (New York: Random House, 1991), 11.
2. Roger Cole, Ph.D., personal communication with author, 3 August 1994.

Chapter 18

1. "The Health Benefits of Small Pleasures," *Glamour,* January 1995, 92.

ABOUT THE AUTHOR

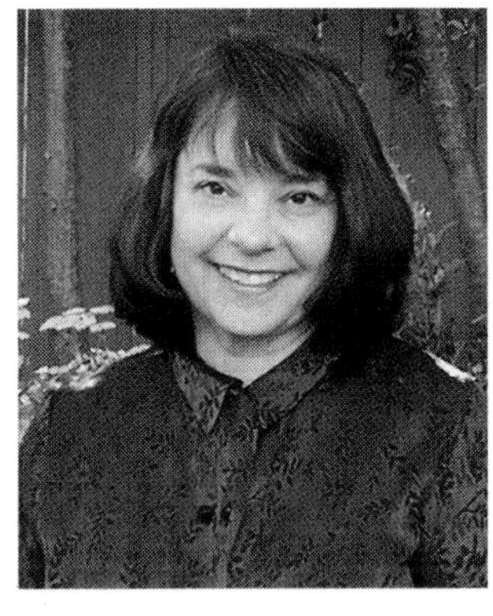

A YOGA TEACHER SINCE 1971, Judith Hanson Lasater holds a bachelor of science degree in physical therapy from the University of California, San Francisco, as well as a doctorate in East-West psychology from the California Institute of Integral Studies. In 1974 she helped found the Institute for Yoga Teacher Education (now the Iyengar Institute of San Francisco), a nationally known yoga teacher training program that has since trained thousands of teachers. In 1975 she cofounded *Yoga Journal* magazine. Judith modeled yoga poses for *Yoga Journal* and started and served on its editorial advisory board. She created and wrote the asana column in the magazine for thirteen years, as well as dozens of other articles relating to postures, anatomy, kinesiology, yoga therapeutics, breathing exercises, and the psychology and philosophy of yoga.

She is president of the California Yoga Teachers Association, the oldest independent professional yoga teachers' association in the United States. She has served on the advisory boards of the International Yoga Studies Association, the medical journal *Alternative Therapies*, and the national registry association for yoga teachers, Yoga Alliance.

Judith has taught yoga as an invited teacher at national and international conventions of yoga teachers for decades. For three years she was a featured speaker at the Governor's Women's Conference in Long Beach, CA, and was twice the opening keynote speaker at *Yoga Journal*'s annual yoga conference. She has also been a speaker at the IDEA-*Yoga Journal* Conference in Anaheim, CA, the Yoga Northwest Conference, the Kripalu Conscious Parenting Conference, and the Yoga in Toronto Conference. Judith was featured in the fortieth anniversary issue of *Natural Heath* magazine as one of the six leaders in the natural health field in the United States.

She has trained beginning students and teachers alike in asana, pranayama (breathing), meditation, anatomy, kinesiology, yoga therapeutics, yoga philosophy, and restorative yoga, one of her specialties. She teaches in San Francisco as well as across the United States and throughout the world. During her second visit to Russia, she directed the production of a video on therapeutic yoga to be used in Russian military hospitals. She has also been an invited guest teacher for the heart patients in Dr. Dean Ornish's Preventative Health program for heart disease as well as in his prostate study using yoga. In 2007 she was an invited speaker at UC Davis School of Medicine, under the auspices of the Complimentary and Alternative Medicine Program.

Judith is the author of:

Living Your Yoga (2000)
30 Essential Yoga Poses (2003)
Yoga for Pregnancy (2004)
Yoga Abs (2005)
A Year of Living Your Yoga (2006)
Yogabody (2009)
What We Say Matters (2009)
Relax and Renew (2nd edition, 2011)

Judith has served as an advisor for a National Institutes of Health (NIH) project studying the effects of yoga on lower back pain for the Osher Center for Integrative Medicine, as well as a consultant on another NIH project on chronic obstructive pulmonary disease (COPD) with the University of San Francisco. She recently completed advising an NIH study using restorative yoga to reduce hot flashes and is consulting on two other NIH studies, one on pregnancy and restorative yoga and another on restorative yoga for reducing anxiety for participants in drug rehabilitation.

She lives in the San Francisco Bay Area. For more information about her yoga classes and teleclasses, workshops, retreats, and teacher trainings, visit www.judithlasater.com and www.restorativeyogateachers.com.

ABOUT THE MODELS

THERESA ELLIOTT is the director of Taj Yoga, in Seattle, WA. She began her yoga study in 1987 and was certified to teach in 1990. Theresa modeled for the photographs in Judith Hanson Lasater's *30 Essential Yoga Poses* and is the cover model of the second edition of *Relax and Renew.*

CAROL NELSON has been studying and teaching yoga since the mid 1970s. She is Teacher-in-Residence at Windows to Sea on Martha's Vineyard, which offers small group classes, private sessions, and workshops with internationally known guest teachers.

RICHARD ROSEN has been a student of yoga since 1980 and a teacher since 1986. He is the director of the Piedmont Yoga Studio, in Oakland, CA. Richard is the author of several books, including *The Yoga of Breath,* and is a contributor to *Yoga Journal.*

CAROL WONG is a physical therapist in the San Francisco Bay Area, where she lives with her husband, David Berger, and son Adam. These photographs were taken in the twenty-ninth week of her second pregnancy.

INDEX